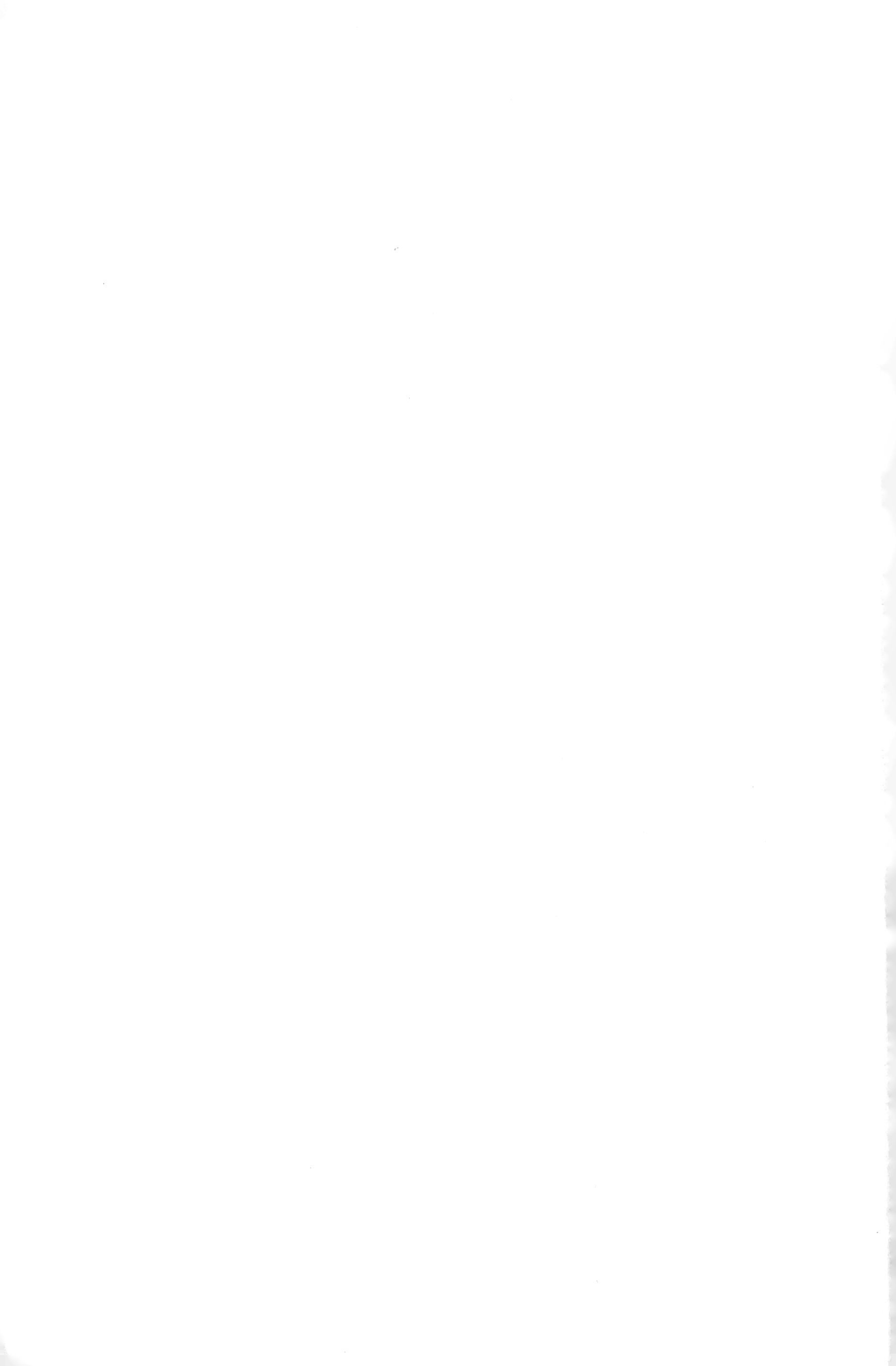

Handbook of
DERMATOLOGY TREATMENTS

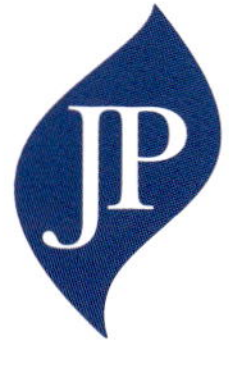

A practical guide to topical treatments, systemic therapies and procedural dermatology

Handbook of
DERMATOLOGY
TREATMENTS

Michael Ardern-Jones BSc MBBS DPhil FRCP
Associate Professor of Dermatology
University of Southampton
Southampton, UK

Philip Hampton PhD MBBS BMedSci FRCP
Consultant Dermatologist
Newcastle Hospitals NHS Trust
Newcastle, UK

Ruth Ann Vleugels MD MPH
Associate Professor
Harvard Medical School
Brigham and Women's Hospital
Boston, USA

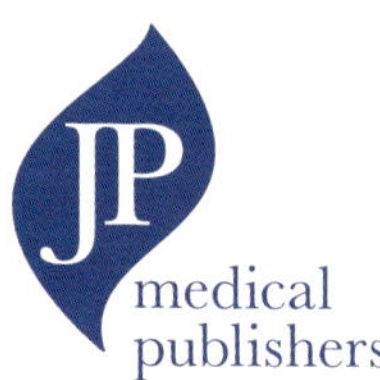

JP
medical publishers

London • Panama City • New Delhi

British Library Cataloguing in Publication Data
A catalogue record for this book is available from the British Library

Library of Congress Cataloging in Publication Data
A catalog record for this book is available from the Library of Congress

Publisher:	Richard Furn
Associate Publisher:	Sue Hodgson
Development Editors:	Gavin Smith, Alison Whitehouse
Editorial Assistant:	Katie Pattullo
Design:	Designers Collective Ltd

Preface

At any one time, skin disease affects almost one third of the world's population. Physically, the result is derangement of one or more functions of the skin, such as regulation of fluid balance, temperature control and immunologic responses. Psychologically, the impact of changes in appearance of the skin can be profound. Along with the significant variation in skin structure in different body sites (including hair and nails), these factors produce significant variation in the clinical presentation, course and severity of skin diseases. To be optimal, management has to be precisely tailored for the disease and the patient's condition, and clinicians therefore require a wide knowledge of the therapeutic options in order to make the best prescribing decisions. *Handbook of Dermatology Treatments* provides that knowledge.

Keeping up to date has two facets: treatments are constantly evolving and over time the demand or need for them changes. An example of the latter is the increasing prevalence of skin cancer in fair-skinned populations, which has resulted in an increased demand for surgical dermatology. On the former topic, clinicians must be aware not only of the latest topical and systemic products but also of increasingly complex new management approaches. In the era of targeted biologic therapies, greater expertise is now required in managing inflammatory cutaneous diseases, for example.

Handbook of Dermatology Treatments was conceived with the busy healthcare practitioner in mind. There are many texts which focus on the clinical presentation of skin disease and the approach to diagnosis but few offer a clear account of how to prescribe. To address that deficit, this book is a comprehensive overview of management options specific to dermatology. Considerations before prescribing, including potential adverse effects, choice of dose and, where necessary, monitoring and follow-up are all covered. Practical descriptions of dermatologic techniques are included.

In choosing which treatments to include, we have aimed for a list which all experienced skin care professionals should be familiar with. We recognize that this book will be referred to in many regions of the world, where prescribing regulations vary. Accordingly, we have made the information compatible with both US and European regulations, in the knowledge that this will make it generally applicable more widely. In writing for a global community, safety during pregnancy and lactation is the most challenging area: while we have identified medications universally recognized to be potentially harmful, we advise readers to remember different regulatory authorities take different approaches and to consult their local formulary for advice.

We trust our target audience of dermatologists, primary care practitioners and specialist nurses will find this book helpful in their management of patients with skin diseases.

Michael Ardern-Jones
Philip Hampton
Ruth Ann Vleugels
March 2017

Contents

Topical treatments

Systemic therapies

Procedural dermatology

Acknowledgements

This book would not have been possible without the generous help of our chapter authors, all of whom are colleagues and friends. We are incredibly grateful to all of them and for their tolerance of our revisions to their text. Thanks must go also to our patients who generously allowed us to photograph their conditions as illustrations for the chapters.

We are grateful to Gavin Smith, Katie Pattullo, Richard Furn and Sue Hodgson at JP Medical who have taken this book from its inception to publication.

Finally, special thanks to our families who have had to put up with the evenings and weekends absorbed by the construction of this text.

MAJ
PH
RAV
March 2017

Contributors

Milan Anadkat MD
Biologic therapy: for melanoma and BCC
Associate Professor of Dermatology
Washington University School of Medicine
St Louis, MO
USA

Michael Ardern-Jones BSc MBBS DPhil FRCP
Antifungal agents
Associate Professor of Dermatology
University of Southampton
Southampton
UK

Antoni Azón MD PhD
Liquid nitrogen
Triamcinolone (intralesional)
Professor of Dermatology
University Hospital Sant Joan
Rovira I Virgili University
Reus
Spain

Antoni Bennàssar Vicens MD PhD
Biopsy (incisional)
Consultant Dermatologist
Hospital Clínic of Barcelona
Barcelona
Spain

John Berth-Jones FRCP
Corticosteroids
Tars
Consultant Dermatologist
University Hospital
Coventry
UK

David Brass MBChB
Surgical complications (management)
Consultant Dermatologist and Mohs Surgeon
Royal Victoria Infirmary
Newcastle upon Tyne
UK

Sara Brown BSc MBChB MD FRCPE
Corticosteroids
Emollients
Professor of Molecular and Genetic Dermatology
Ninewells Hospital and Medical School
Dundee
UK

Jeff Callen MD
Azathioprine
Mycophenolate mofetil
Professor of Medicine (Dermatology)
University of Louisville School of Medicine
Louisville, KY
USA

Alex Chamberlain MBBS (Hons) FACD
Imiquimod
Consultant Dermatologist
Glenferrie Dermatology
Malvern
Australia

Hywel Cooper MRCP BM BMedSci IntDipAcu
Glucocorticoids
Thalidomide
Dermatology Consultant
St Mary's Hospital
Portsmouth
UK

Susan M Cooper MD FRCP MRCGP
Dressings and bandages
Consultant Dermatologist
Oxford University Hospitals Foundation Trust
Oxford
UK

Daniela Cunha MD
Curettage
Consultant Dermatologist and Mohs Surgeon
Hospital CUF Descobertas
Lisbon
Portugal

Emily E G Davies BMedSci BMBS MRCP
Dressings and bandages
Consultant Dermatologist
Department of Dermatology
Gloucestershire Hospitals NHS Foundation Trust
Gloucester
UK

Scott A Elman MD
Isotretinoin
Resident in Internal Medicine and Dermatology
Harvard Combined Residency Program in Medicine and Dermatology
Harvard University
Boston, MA
USA

Peter Farr MD FRCP
Phototherapy
Sunscreens
Consultant Dermatologist
Professor of Clinical Photobiology
Royal Victoria Infirmary
Newcastle upon Tyne
UK

Alisa Femia MD
Intravenous immunoglobulin
Methotrexate
Assistant Professor
The Ronald O. Perelman Department of Dermatology
New York University School of Medicine
New York, NY
USA

Nicole Fett MD MSCE
Calcineurin inhibitors
Associate Professor of
Dermatology
Oregon Health and Science
University
Portland, OR
USA

**Adam Fityan BM BSc(Hons)
MRCP(UK)**
Hydroxyurea (hydroxycarbamide)
Anti-androgens
Consultant Dermatologist
University Hospital
Southampton NHS Foundation
Trust
Southampton
UK

Sarah Gee MD
Antiseptics
Antiparasitic agents
Dermatologist
Vitalogy Skincare
Austin, TX
USA

Charlotte Goodhead MBBS
Depigmenting agents
Specialty Registrar in
Dermatology
Royal Victoria infirmary
Newcastle upon Tyne
UK

Clive Grattan MA MD FRCP
*Antihistamines, sodium
cromoglicate and leukotriene
receptor antagonists*
Consultant Dermatologist
St John's Institute of
Dermatology
Guy's and St Thomas' NHS
Foundation Trust
London
UK

Richard Groves FRCP
Cyclophosphamide
Consultant Dermatologist
St John's Institute of
Dermatology
Guy's and St Thomas' NHS
Foundation Trust
London
UK

**Philip Hampton PhD MBBS
BMedSci FRCP**
Biologic therapy: rituximab
Depigmenting agents
Iontophoresis
Fumaric acid esters (fumarates)
Consultant Dermatologist
Newcastle Hospitals NHS Trust
Newcastle upon Tyne
UK

**Shannon Harrison MBBS MMed
FACD**
Imiquimod
Honorary Clinical Lecturer
Department of Medicine
University of Melbourne
Australia

**Roderick J Hay MD FRCP
FRCPath**
Antifungal agents
Professor of Cutaneous Infection
Kings College Hospital NHS
Trust
London
UK

Meghan Heberton MD
*Biologic therapy: for melanoma
and BCC*
Dermatology Resident
Division of Dermatology
Washington University in St
Louis
St Louis, MO
USA

**Eleanor Higgins MBBCh BAO
MRCPI MScMedEd**
Biologic therapy: for psoriasis
Consultant Dermatologist
St John's Institute of
Dermatology
Guy's and St Thomas'
NHS Foundation Trust
London
UK

Jonathan D Ho MBBS MSc
Colchicine
International Dermatopathology
Fellow
Boston University School of
Medicine
Boston, MA
USA

Sarah Hahn Hsu MD
Colchicine
Cosmetic Dermatologic Surgery
Fellow
Maryland Laser Skin and Vein
Institute
Baltimore, MD
USA

Sotonye Imadojemu MD MBE
Cyclosporine (ciclosporin)
Antimalarials
Chief Resident, Internal
Medicine and Dermatology
Hospital of the University of
Pennsylvania
Philadelphia, PA
USA

**Zarif Jabbar-Lopez MA MSci
MBBS MPH MRCP**
Fumaric acid esters (fumarates)
NIHR Academic Clinical Fellow
Royal Victoria Infirmary
Newcastle upon Tyne
UK

H Ray Jalian MD
Depilatory treatments
Laser therapy
Health Sciences Assistant
Clinical Professor
UCLA Division of Dermatology
Los Angeles, CA
USA

**Nicole Kelleners-Smeets MD
PhD**
Excisions
Dermatologist
Maastricht University Medical
Centre
Maastricht
Netherlands

Amina Khalid MBBS MRCP
DermDipGlas SCEDerm
Emollients
Corticosteroids
Specialist Registrar in
Dermatology
Ninewells Hospital and Medical
school
Dundee
UK

Christina Lam MD
Colchicine
Dapsone and sulfapyridine
Assistant Professor of
Dermatology
Boston University School of
Medicine
Boston, MA
USA

James A Langtry MBBS MRCP
Mohs micrographic surgery
*Surgical complications
(management)*
Consultant Dermatologist
Royal Victoria Infirmary
Newcastle upon Tyne
UK

Alison Layton MB ChB FRCP
Antibiotics for acne
Consultant Dermatologist
Harrogate and District NHS
Foundation Trust
Harrogate
UK

Eglantine Lebas MD
Scabicides
Clinical Fellow in
Dermatopathology
St John's Institute of
Dermatology
Guy's and St Thomas' NHS
Foundation Trust
London
UK

**Tabi A Leslie BSc(Hons) MBBS
FRCP(Lon)**
*Antihistamines, sodium
cromoglicate and leukotriene
receptor antagonists*
Consultant Dermatologist
Royal Free Hospital
London
UK

Daniel Mazori MD
Intravenous immunoglobulin
Dermatology Resident
State University of New York
Downstate Medical Center
New York, NY
USA

Mariah N Mason MD PhD
Calcineurin inhibitors
Dermatologist
Northwest – Kaiser Permanente
Portland, OR
USA

Elena M Mercedé MD
Biopsy (incisional)
Consultant Dermatologist
Hospital Clínic in Barcelona
Barcelona
Spain

Tiago Mestre MD
Curettage
Dermatologist and Mohs
Surgeon
Royal Victoria Infirmary
Newcastle upon Tyne
UK

Charles Mitchell MBBS, MRCP
Glucocorticoids
Thalidomide
Dermatologist
St Mary's Hospital
Portsmouth Hospitals NHS Trust
Portsmouth
UK

Caroline Morgan DM FRCP
Anti-actinic therapies
Retinoids
Consultant Dermatologist
Poole Hospital NHS Trust
Poole
UK

Colin A Morton MB ChB MD
Photodynamic therapy
Consultant Dermatologist
Stirling Community Hospital
Stirling
UK

Samuel L Moschella MD
Acitretin
Alitretinoin
Senior Dermatologic Consultant
Lahey Hospital & Medical Center
Burlington, MA
USA

Vinod Nambudiri MD MBA
Acitretin
Alitretinoin
Attending Physician
Brigham and Women's Hospital
Boston, MA
USA

Michelle Oakford MBBS FRCP
Keratolytics
Consultant Dermatologist
Royal South Hants Hospital
Southampton
UK

**Thomas Oliphant
MBBCh(Hons) BSc MRCP**
Mohs micrographic surgery
Consultant Dermatologist/Mohs
Surgeon
Royal Victoria Infirmary
Newcastle upon Tyne
UK

**Ursula B M Quinn MBBCh BAO
MRCP(UK)**
Retinoids
Specialty Trainee in
Dermatology
Poole Hospital NHS Foundation
Trust
Poole
UK

**Nick J Reynolds BSc MBBS MD
FRCP**
Dithranol
Vitamin D analogs
Consultant Dermatologist
Institute of Cellular Medicine
Newcastle University Medical
School
Newcastle upon Tyne
UK

Misha Rosenbach MD
Antimalarials
Cyclosporine (ciclosporin)
Assistant Professor of
Dermatology & Internal
Medicine
Perelman School of Medicine
University of Pennsylvania
Philadelphia, PA
USA

Suzanne Sachsman MD
Antiseptics
Antiparasitic agents
Resident in Dermatology
Division of Dermatology
University of California Los
Angeles
Los Angeles, CA
USA

Edward Seaton DM FRCP
Acne and rosacea treatments
Honorary Consultant
Dermatologist
Royal Free Hospital
London
UK

Kate Short BSc DTM&H FRCP
*Antibiotics for cutaneous
infections*
Antibiotics for skin infections
Consultant Dermatologist
The Royal Victoria Infirmary
Newcastle upon Tyne
UK

**Tee Wei Siah MBChB
MRCP(Derm)**
*Sensitizing agents
(diphencyprone)*
Minoxidil
Consultant Dermatologist
Royal Victoria Infirmary
Newcastle upon Tyne
UK

**Catherine H Smith MD MRCP
FRCP**
Biologic therapy: for psoriasis
Professor of Dermatology and
Therapeutics
St John's Institute of
Dermatology
Guy's and St Thomas' NHS
Foundation Trust
London
UK

**Jane Sterling MB BChir MA
FRCP PhD**
*Antivirals: acyclovir and
penciclovir*
Antiviral agents
Consultant Dermatologist
Addenbrooke's Hospital
Cambridge
UK

Hillary Tsibris MD
Antiperspirants
Botulinum toxin
Instructor in Dermatology
Harvard Medical School
Boston, MA
USA

Rachel L V Waas MBChB MRCP
*Surgical complications
(management)*
Specialty Trainee in
Dermatology
Royal Victoria Infirmary
Newcastle upon Tyne
UK

**Stephen L Walker PhD
MRCP(UK) DTM&H**
Scabicides
Senior Lecturer
London School of Hygiene and
Tropical Medicine
London
UK

**Keith C P Wu MA BM BCh PhD
MRCP**
Vitamin D analogs
Specialty Registrar in
Dermatology
Royal Victoria Infirmary
Newcastle upon Tyne
UK

Fei-Shiuann Clarissa Yang MD
Botulinum toxin
Antiperspirants
Outpatient Clinical Director
Brigham and Women's Hospital
Boston, MA
USA

Topical treatments

Acne and rosacea treatments

Dermatologic indications

- *Licensed indications:* topical benzoyl peroxide, azelaic acid, clindamycin, and erythromycin are licensed for acne and rosacea. Topical ivermectin, metronidazole, and brimonidine are licensed for rosacea
- *Other common indications:* topical erythromycin is used for erythrasma and pitted keratolysis, topical clindamycin for hidradenitis suppurativa, retinoids for acne and anti-aging treatment

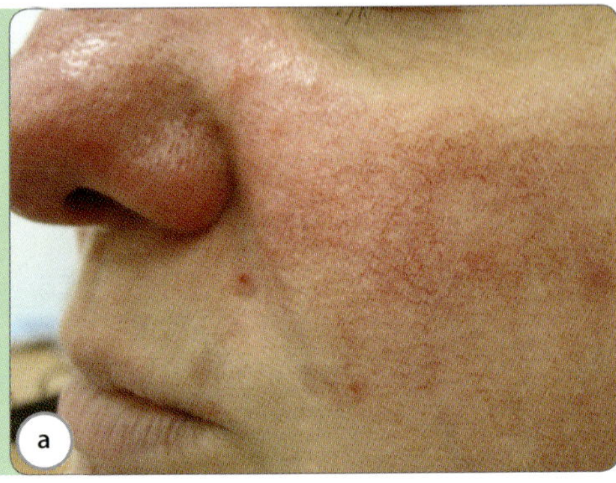

Background

Acne

Acne is almost universally prevalent in adolescence, but can occur at any age and is particularly common in adult women. Excessive production of sebum (oil), keratinocyte proliferation blocking the pilosebaceous duct, and bacterial colonization of the follicle (*Propionibacterium acnes*) are some of the factors that induce acne.

Acne causes comedones (black- and whiteheads) as well as inflammatory papules and pustules on the face and upper trunk. Acne may cause scarring in genetically prone individuals.

Rosacea

Rosacea commonly develops during early to mid adult life and is more common in individuals with fair complexions and long-term, excessive sun exposure. Vasomotor dysregulation occurs, causing facial flushing that lasts many minutes. With time, fixed erythema and visible telangiectases develop.

Rosacea subtypes

Erythemato-telangiectatic rosacea: facial redness, flushing, and few inflammatory lesions

Papulopustular rosacea: more inflammatory lesions along with redness

Dermatologic prescribing

Acne

- In acne, benzoyl peroxide, clindamycin, and erythromycin kill or inhibit *P. acnes*; retinoids and azelaic acid inhibit comedone formation; and antibiotics, retinoids, and azelaic acid have additional anti-inflammatory effects. These are often more effective when used in combination than as single agents
- Once daily application of benzoyl peroxide 2.5% is as effective as 10% but is much less irritating

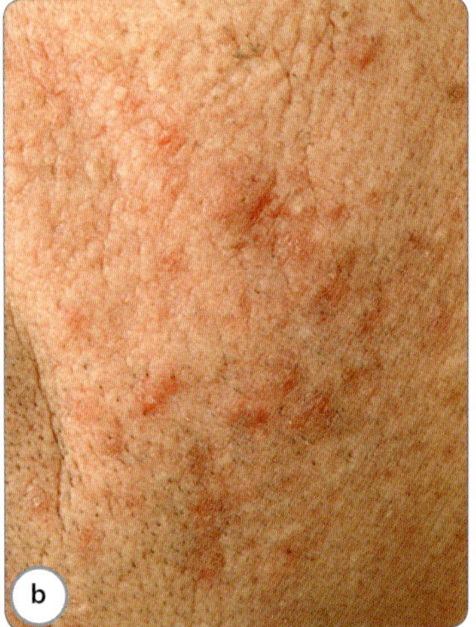

Figure 1.1 The chronic inflammation of rosacea (a) can lead to the development of telangiectasia. Once present, telangiectases can only be removed by intense pulsed light (IPL) or laser treatment (b).

- Topical retinoids should be used in the majority of acne patients because they inhibit development of new lesions. Retinoids need to be applied at night and should not be used in pregnancy
- In order to avoid the development of bacterial antibiotic resistance, topical erythromycin and clindamycin should not be used as single agents. Instead they can be used in combination with benzoyl peroxide or topical retinoids
- Azelaic acid 15–20% once daily is helpful in patients who develop post-inflammatory hyperpigmentation following acne lesions (especially in Asian or Afro-Caribbean skin types), because it inhibits pigment production

Rosacea

- In papulopustular rosacea, topical metronidazole (1–2 times daily), azelaic acid 15% (1–2 times daily), and ivermectin (at night) are highly effective. Topical ivermectin appears to be superior to topical metronidazole and kills *Demodex* mites, which are found at higher levels in patients with rosacea although their pathogenic role is unknown. These treatments are ineffective in erythemato-telangectatic rosacea

- Brimonidine gel is a vasoconstrictor and reduces facial redness for up to 12–16 hours per application. Treatment can be applied each morning or it may be used as required 30–60 minutes before social engagements to control facial erythema

- Erythema and persistent telangiectasia may respond to IPL or pulsed dye laser

Common problems

- Topical treatments commonly cause skin irritation (reduce amount and/or frequency of application)

- Benzoyl peroxide can bleach fabric. Patients should be warned to use white bedding and towels

- Some rosacea patients find that topical applications cause stinging

- Rosacea patients trying brimonidine gel should be warned that they may experience rebound flushing as the therapeutic effect wears off. This side effect often limits its use in these patients

- Topical treatment failure may warrant combination with oral treatments in patients with acne and papulopustular rosacea

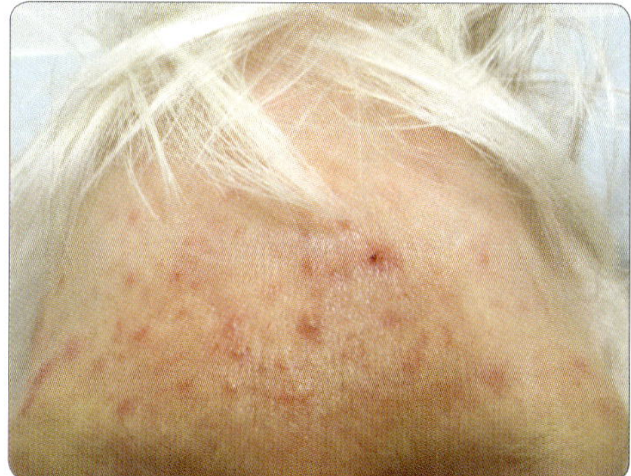

Figure 1.2 The cheeks and nose are the most common sites for papules and pustules in rosacea but the forehead and more peripheral areas can also be affected.

Treatment pearls

- Careful counselling of patients is essential to success of treatment. Benzoyl peroxide or topical retinoids commonly cause the skin to become inflamed after a few days. Often, patients are counselled to start these topical therapies two to three times weekly and then increase treatment frequency as tolerated to improve tolerability and compliance. Most patients can use treatments daily, although some can only do so every 2–3 days, which is still effective

- Patients should be advised to treat the entire affected area and not to apply treatments only to their active lesions

- Both acne and rosacea patients will benefit from use of non-comedogenic moisturizers. Paraffin-based moisturizers such as aqueous creams should be avoided because they are comedogenic

- Rosacea patients should be encouraged to wear high-factor, broad-spectrum sunscreens

- Use of topical treatments containing combinations of two different acne treatments is often more practical for patients

- Rosacea often co-exists with seborrheic dermatitis. If the scalp is inflamed or the face scaly, consider the addition of ketoconazole shampoo to the scalp and/or face twice weekly, rinsing after 3–5 minutes. Topical calcineurin inhibitors may be helpful for concomitant facial seborrheic dermatitis, as facial application of topical steroids should be avoided in patients with rosacea

- Most treatments (with the exception of brimonidine) take several weeks to work. Reassessing patients after 8 weeks is reasonable

Further reading

Thiboutot D, Gollnick H, Bettoli, et al. New insights into the management of acne: An update from the Global Alliance to Improve Outcomes in Acne group. J Am Acad Dermatol 2009; 60: 1–50.

van Zuuren EJ, Fedorowicz Z, Carter B, et al. Treatments for rosacea. Cochrane Database Syst Rev 2015: CD003262.

Anti-actinic therapies

Dermatologic indications

- *5-fluorouracil (5-FU):* actinic keratoses and pre-cancerous field change, squamous cell carcinoma in situ (Bowen's disease), superficial basal cell carcinoma

- *Diclofenac 3% gel:* actinic keratoses and pre-cancerous field change

- *Ingenol mebutate 0.05% and 0.015%:* actinic keratoses and pre-cancerous field change

- Imiquimod may also be used (see **Chapter 14**)

- 5-fluorouracil and salicylic acid combination (5-FU/SA) can also be used to treat viral warts

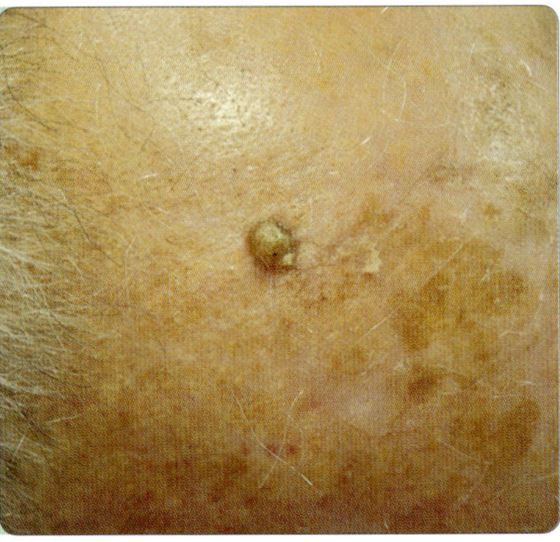

Figure 2.1 Hyperkeratotic actinic keratosis on the scalp with surrounding field change.

Background

Actinic keratoses (AK) are intra-epithelial proliferations of atypical keratinocytes found in the epidermis. Approximately 10% of affected individuals will develop squamous cell carcinoma of the skin within 10 years. AKs are very common, particularly in patients with light skin. In the UK, for example, 34% of men and 18% of women aged over 70 years have actinic keratoses.

AKs typically present as skin-colored to erythematous scaly macules, papules, or thin plaques. Lesion size ranges from a few millimeters up to 2 cm. They are caused by chronic, cumulative sun exposure.

Lesions may be single or multiple (pre-cancerous field change refers to a wider area affected by numerous areas of AKs).

Organ transplant patients have a 250-fold higher risk of developing actinic keratoses.

Dermatologic prescribing

- There are numerous therapeutic approaches to treat AKs, including ablative procedures (cryotherapy, curettage, laser) to mainly treat individual lesions, and topical treatments (5% fluorouracil, diclofenac gel, ingenol mebutate, imiquimod, and photodynamic therapy) directed at treating both individual lesions and field change

- It is important to select the most appropriate treatment. Focal ablative procedures will not prevent new lesions from appearing in adjacent dysplastic tissue. Topical agents can treat larger areas. A combination of both strategies should be considered

- 5-fluorouracil application regimens vary but include twice a day for 3 weeks, once daily for 4 weeks, or on alternate days for 8 weeks. Localized skin inflammation is usually evident during the second or third week of therapy

- 5-FU/SA is licensed for individual actinic keratosis therapy. The lotion is painted onto the skin at night, producing a film that is peeled off the following morning. Treatment is once a day for up to 12 weeks. 3% diclofenac gel is used twice a day for 12 weeks. It causes less skin inflammation and is therefore less effective at clearing actinic damage than the other topical therapies reviewed here

- Topical ingenol mebutate is produced in two strengths: 0.015% for 3 days for the head and neck and 0.05% for 2 days for the trunk and limbs. It covers an area of actinic damage up to 25 cm^2. Compliance is high due to the short duration of treatment

- Topical diclofenac is available as 3% gel to apply twice daily for 60–90 days. It should be applied thinly; maximum 8 g per day. Although topical diclofenac produces less of an inflammatory response, the efficacy of this treatment is lower.

- Cryotherapy is also a useful treatment option (see **Chapter 53**)

- Photodynamic therapy and currettage may also be considered in selected cases (see **Chapters 55** and **57**)

Cautions

- All topical treatments for actinic damage are expected to cause localized erythema, edema, and sometimes superficial blistering, erosions,

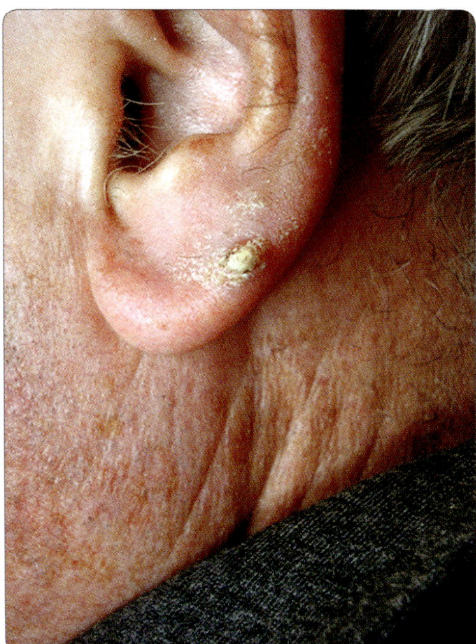

Figure 2.2 Hyperkeratotic actinic keratosis on the ear. Histological analysis may be required to distinguish from squamous cell carcinoma.

and crusting of the skin. The severity of the reaction varies between patients, the body site treated, and the particular topical therapy selected

- Careful patient education is needed at all times, particularly if these treatments are to be used close to the eye

- The US FDA has recently warned about the increased risk of severe allergic reactions and herpes zoster infections with the use of ingenol mebutate. Patients should also be advised to avoid applying the gel in, near, and around the mouth, lips and eye area

Common problems

- The irritant skin reaction peaks at day 4 for ingenol mebutate and after 2–3 weeks of treatment with 5-fluorouracil

- Patients need to avoid direct sunlight during the treatment period and use high factor sunscreen for at least 3 months post-treatment

- All topical actinic therapies can cause phototoxicity and contact dermatitis

Treatment pearls

- Compliance will be improved if patients are shown photographs of the possible reactions they may experience

- Topical 1% hydrocortisone or another low potency topical corticosteroid applied after the completed course of 5-fluorouracil twice daily for 2 weeks will shorten and lessen any irritant reaction. There is little or no benefit in applying topical corticosteroid after ingenol or diclofenac treatment. Simple bland emollients such as petroleum jelly will suffice

- Any AKs that persist after field directed therapy may respond to cryotherapy or 5-FU/SA

- Complete clearance of lesions can be delayed several weeks beyond completion of topical therapies

- A diagnosis of squamous cell carcinoma should be considered in those lesions that are rapidly growing, tender with an indurated base, or do not respond to topical treatment

- The use of high factor (30+) sunscreen should be encouraged, along with self-monitoring and early detection of lesions

- 5-FU under occlusion can result in an up to 95% clearance rate for common viral warts

- Severe reactions with the use of fluoruracil topical cream, especially those including systemic effects, should prompt the physician to consider dihydropyrimidine dehydrogenase (DPD) enzyme deficiency. Individuals with DPD deficiency should not use fluoruracil topically (or systemically)

Further reading

Bower C, Keohane S, Kownacki S, et al. PCDS Guidelines: Actinic (Solar) Keratosis – Primary Care Treatment Pathway. Hatfield, UK: Primary Care Dermatology Society, 2014.

De Berker D, McGregor JM, Hughes BR. British Association of Dermatologists Therapy Guidelines and Audit Subcommittee. Guidelines for the management of actinic keratoses. Br J Dermatol 2007; 156:222–230.

Dodson JM, DeSpain J, Hewett JE, Clark DP. Malignant potential of actinic keratoses and the controversy over treatment. A patient-orientated perspective. Arch Dermatol 1991; 127:1029–1031.

Antibiotics for cutaneous infections

Dermatologic indications

- Superficial bacterial skin infections
- Prevention of infection after surgery or injury
- Impetigo
- Secondarily infected eczema
- Burns
- Adjunctive therapy in leg ulcers

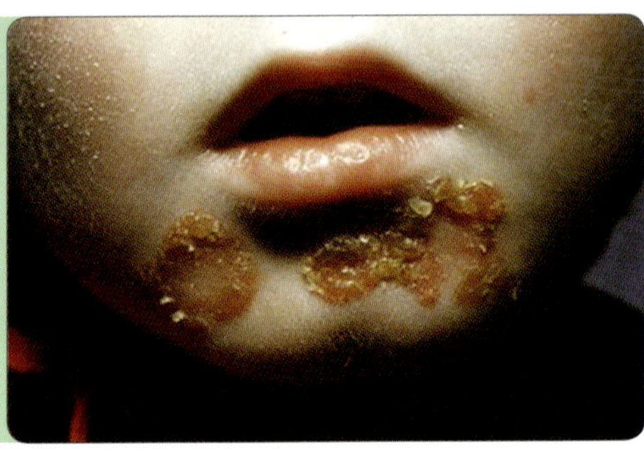

Figure 3.1 Impetigo on the chin of a child. Note the classical 'golden crust' of *S. aureus*.

Background

Bacterial infections of the skin are very common and account for approximately 20% of patients seen in dermatology clinics. They are characterized by redness, crusting, oozing, and pustulation.

Not all skin conditions that are red, crusted, oozing, or pustular are infected. A number of cutaneous diseases can present with non-infectious pustular inflammation. It is therefore critical to take bacterial cultures in order to guide therapeutic management.

Superficial bacterial infections can affect any body site.

Dermatologic prescribing

Fusidic acid

- A narrow spectrum antibacterial used to treat staphylococcal skin infections. When used in combination with topical corticosteroids, it can be very useful in the treatment of secondarily infected eczema

Mupirocin

- Clinically active against staphylococci, streptococci (groups A, B, C, and G) and some Gram-negative anaerobic bacteria. The intranasal preparation, Bactroban is used to eradicate nasopharyngeal carriage of *Staphylococcus aureus* (including MRSA). Bactroban nasal ointment should be used with caution in patients with moderate or severe renal impairment as it contains polyethylene glycol

- Used to treat methicillin-resistant *S. aureus*. In adults and children over one year, it is typically applied up to three times daily. Duration is usually 5 days for decolonization and 5-10 days for treatment of impetigo

Neomycin

- Effective against Gram-positive and Gram-negative bacteria including *S. aureus*, *Escherichia coli*, *Haemophilus influenzae*, *Proteus* spp, and *Serratia* spp. It is generally not effective against *Pseudomonas aeruginosa*

- Usually applied up to three times daily

- Most common side effects are erythema, pruritus, and edema

- Uncommon side effects including ototoxicity, nephrotoxicity and neuromuscular blockade have been reported after application of neomycin, especially in patients undergoing irrigation of wounds or surgical sites or those receiving treatment for skin ulcers, burns or extensive areas of denuded skin

Polymyxin B

- Used to treat a number of Gram-negative organisms including *P. aeruginosa*, *E. coli*, *Klebsiella pneumoniae*, *Enterobacteria aerogenes*, *H. Influenzae*, *Proteus mirabilis*, and *Serratia marcescens*. It is also effective for multi drug resistant (MDR) Gram-negative bacteria. It is not active against Gram-positive organisms

- Typically applied twice daily

Polyfax (polmyxin B plus bacitracin)

- Polyfax is an ointment that is effective against Gram-positive and Gram-negative bacteria

- It is sometimes used for secondary intention healing following skin cancer surgery

Silver sulfadiazine

- Commonly used:

- as prophylaxis and treatment of infection in burns (applied daily or more frequently if wound is very exudative, i.e if the tissues are bathed in fluid)

- as an adjunct to short term treatment of infection in leg ulcers and pressure sores (applied daily or on alternate days but not recommended if the ulcer is very exudative, i.e if the tissues are bathed in fluid)

- as an adjunct to prophylaxis of infection in skin grafts and for conservative management of finger-tip injuries (applied every two to three days)
- When used in conjunction with cimetidine, there is an increased risk of leukopenia
- It is the active ingredient in Flamazine cream
- It is contraindicated in patients with a history of sensitivity to sulfonamides and should be used cautiously in patients with G6PD deficiency, renal or hepatic disease, or porphyria. Localized argyria due to deposits of silver in the dermis may also occur

Common problems

- To minimize the development of resistant organisms, it is advisable to limit the choice of topical antibiotics to those not being used systemically
- Some topical antibiotics (e.g. neomycin) can cause sensitization and can show cross-sensitivity with other aminoglycoside antibiotics such as gentamicin
- Aminoglycosides and polymyxins can cause ototoxicity if used over large areas of skin, particularly in patients with renal impairment, children, and the elderly
- 5–15% of patients using neomycin develop allergic contact dermatitis, especially when applied to ulcerated skin

Treatment pearls

- For uncomplicated impetigo, either topical fusidic acid or mupirocin is as effective, if not more effective, than systemic antibiotics
- Acute impetigo affecting small areas of skin may be treated with short-term topical application of either fusidic acid or mupirocin, usually three to four times daily. If the impetigo is extensive or longstanding (>7 days), an appropriate oral antibiotic should be used
- Topical antibiotics can be used to eradicate wound bacteria prior to skin grafting or for reducing odor associated with non-healing necrotic wounds. Topical antimicrobials (which achieve high local levels) can be added to systemic antibiotics in patients with infected ischemic wounds who are not suitable for revascularization
- Absorption of silver sulfadiazene can rarely lead to skin staining and silver toxicity when used in excess. Therefore, application should be limited in extensive infections or young children

Further reading

Geria AN, Schwartz RA. Impetigo update: new challenges in the era of methicillin resistance. Cutis 2010; 85:65–70.

Hartman-Adams H, Banvard C. Impetigo: diagnosis and treatment. Am Fam Physician 2014; 90:229-35.

McEvoy GK. American hospital formulary service drug information. London: Pharmaceutical Press, 2013.

Antifungal agents

Dermatologic indications

- *Common dermatologic uses:* tinea pedis, tinea corporis, tinea cruris, tinea versicolor (pityriasis versicolor), seborrheic dermatitis, skin infections due to dermatophytes, yeasts (e.g. *Candida* species), molds and other fungi

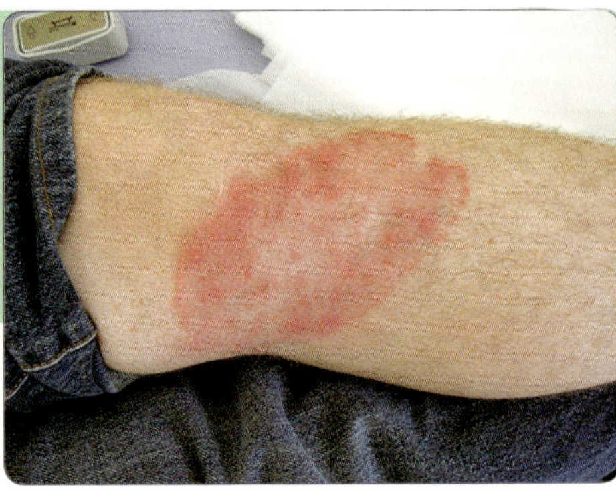

Figure 4.1 Dermatophyte infection of the medial left leg.

Background

Fungal infections of the skin typically present with well-demarcated scaly patches with peripheral induration; occasionally, pustules are present. They are heterogeneous in appearance and should be considered in the differential diagnosis of any inflamed, scaly skin lesions.

Fungal infections causing typical patches on the body are known as tinea corporis or 'ringworm', but infections are not always annular and can present variably as scaly patches or boggy plaques

Fungal infections can affect any body site including the scalp, groin or nails. Interdigital fungal infection of the feet or tinea pedis commonly presents with macerated skin changes, most often between the fourth and fifth web spaces.

Common conditions appropriate for topical therapy include tinea corporis (ringworm), tinea pedis (athlete's foot) and tinea cruris (jock itch).

Fungal infections of the skin are usually caused by dermatophytes or yeasts (e.g. *Candida*), but other organisms such as molds should be considered, especially in toe webs and in nail diseases.

Candida is predominantly a disease of moist surfaces such as the mucosae, groin, skin folds, and nail folds.

Imidazoles (e.g. clotrimazole and miconazole) are effective (fungistatic) against most *Candida* spp and also against *Pityrosporum* yeasts, but less so against dermatophytes. Terbinafine is very effective (fungicidal) against dermatophyte infections but less effective against *Candida*.

Tinea versicolor (pityriasis versicolor) and seborrheic dermatitis involve an inflammatory response to *Malassezia* spp overgrowth, and often respond to anti-yeast therapy (oral or topical)

Dermatologic prescribing

- Topical terbinafine 1% is usually prescribed twice daily for 1–2 weeks
- Topical imidazoles (e.g. clotrimazole, econazole, ketoconazole, and miconazole) are usually prescribed two to three times daily for 1–2 weeks
- Using a combination of imidazoles with other agents, including topical corticosteroids, can speed symptom improvement, but should only be undertaken by those experienced in the management of such conditions
- Products formulated for effective treatment of tinea pedis in one application are available (e.g. Lamisil Once)
- Ketoconazole 2%, zinc pyrithione 1% or selenium sulfide 2.5% shampoos once or twice weekly are useful for seborrheic dermatitis of the scalp and/or face as well as for tinea versicolor (pityriasis versicolor) on the trunk; these medications should be left on for 3–5 minutes prior to rinsing

Common problems

- Treatment of fungal infections of the skin and groin generally requires 2 weeks of therapy, whereas inter-digital fungal infections (tinea pedis or 'athlete's foot') often require 4 weeks of therapy
- Treatment failures often arise when therapy is discontinued too soon. A useful rule is to continue treatment for 1 week after the clinical problem has resolved
- Confirmation of the clinical diagnosis with mycologic sampling is recommended before oral therapy is commenced. Samples should not be collected while topical antifungal medication is being used as this may lead to culture failure. Avoidance of topical treatment for one week is usually adequate to ensure accurate sampling
- Both irritant and allergic contact dermatitis are recognized complications of all topical antifungals

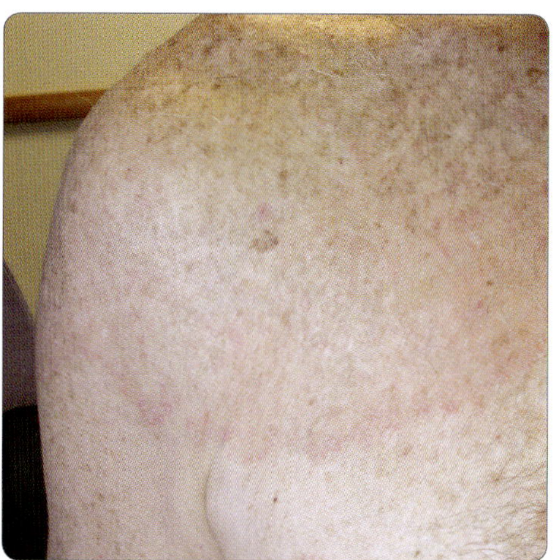

Figure 4.2 Tinea incognito following topical steroid use. Dermatophyte infection of the right upper shoulder. Note the clear cut off between normal and infected skin, with scaling only prominent at the margin.

Further reading

Crawford F, Hollis S. Topical treatments for fungal infections of the skin and nails of the foot. Cochrane Database Syst Rev 2007; 3:CD001434.

El-Gohary M, van Zuuren EJ, Federowizc Z, et al. Topical antifungal treatments for tinea cruris and tinea corporis. Cochrane Database Syst Rev 2014; 8:CD009992.

Kyle AA, Dahl MV. Topical therapy for fungal infections. Am J Clin Dermatol 2004; 5:443–451.

Treatment pearls

- Treatment of tinea pedis requires prevention of a damp environment between the toes. Careful drying after bathing and the use of loose fitting, non-occlusive footwear is beneficial
- Infected socks and footwear can be the cause of recurrent tinea pedis
- Skin absorption of topical antifungals is reduced if clothing is applied immediately following application, as some topical medication will be absorbed into the fibers
- Topical terbinafine has been shown to act more quickly than clotrimazole (1 week versus 4 weeks of treatment)
- Failure of topical antifungal therapy is most commonly due to poor compliance or inappropriate use (e.g. in hairy areas)
- The emollient action of all topical antifungal creams and the antibacterial action of the imidazoles can cause improvement in a variety of non-fungal dermatoses. The response to treatment should therefore not be used as a diagnostic marker of fungal infection
- There is little evidence of differences between imidazoles in terms of efficacy
- Systemic treatment is usually required for more extensive or severe infections
- Non-dermatophyte molds are more frequently found on nails and in toe webs and are usually resistant to standard treatment. They may co-exist with dermatophyte infections
- Some products are also available as sprays for application to larger or hairy areas, but effective treatment of tinea is less reliable with these formulations
- Long-term application of anti-yeast shampoo more than once or twice weekly is likely to have an irritant effect
- The possibility of zoonotic dermatophytes should be considered, particularly in infections of the hand and forearm

Antiperspirants

Dermatologic indications

- Topical aluminum chloride hexahydrate is licensed for hyperhidrosis and is also used for prevention of foot blisters and for aquagenic wrinkling of the palms
- Oral anti-cholinergic drugs used for hyperhidrosis include propantheline bromide oxybutynin and glycopyrronium bromide

Background

Aluminum chloride hexahydrate obstructs the distal eccrine duct and induces atrophy of secretory cells with chronic use.

Propantheline bromide, oxybutynin, and glycopyrronium bromide (glycopyrrolate) are all anticholinergic agents that block muscarinic receptors. The subsequent inhibition of cholinergic signaling in the eccrine glands leads to reduced sweating.

Dermatologic prescribing

Topical

- *Over the counter:* 12% aluminum chloride solution
- *Prescription:* 20% aluminum chloride solution in ethyl alcohol or 15% aluminum chloride in a 2–4% salicylic acid gel
- Aluminum chloride solution should be applied to the affected area nightly for 1–2 weeks and then decreased to one to three times weekly for maintenance therapy. It is important that the skin is completely dry prior to application in order to reduce the risk of irritancy
- Topical application of glycopyrrolate (1–4%) from pre-soaked pads (e.g. Secure wipes) is useful for those intolerant of aluminium chloride and often more effective. Dose titration upwards is recommended because systemic anticholinergic side effects are common even with topical application. Patients should be counseled as to what symptoms to monitor for and advised to reduce application frequency if these side effects are noted

Oral

- Propantheline bromide is licensed to be taken 15 mg three times daily
- The starting dose of glycopyrronium bromide is 1 mg twice daily. The dose may be increased to 1–2 mg two to three times daily if anti-cholinergic side effects allow
- Oxybutynin is prescribed at 5 mg daily, which can be increased to 5 mg twice daily as tolerated if needed

Cautions

- Aluminum chloride hexahydrate:
- *Flammable:* Use caution with electrocautery
- *Pregnancy/lactation:* Safety during pregnancy is unknown. It is classified as probably safe during breast feeding
- Oral anticholinergic drugs share similar side effects. Anecdotal evidence suggests that these are less severe with glycopyrronium bromide
- *Medication interactions:* multiple medication interactions exist, and patients' existing medications should be carefully considered prior to prescribing. Co-administration with tricyclic antidepressants increases anticholinergic effects. Glycopyrrolate increases the effects of digoxin and atenolol and decreases the efficacy of the antipsychotic phenothiazine
- *Ocular:* these should not be used in patients with glaucoma due to increased intraocular pressure
- *Neurologic:* these are contraindicated in patients with myasthenia gravis
- *Gastrointestinal:* these are contraindicated in patients with paralytic ileus or pyloric stenosis due to decreased gastric motility
- *Genitourinary:* use with caution in patients with urinary outflow tract obstruction due to urinary hesitancy
- *Pregnancy/lactation:* Safety in pregnancy is dependent upon the oral agent, with the safest is considered to be oxybutynin

Common problems

Aluminum chloride hexahydrate

- Irritant contact dermatitis associated with application site burning and tingling can occur

Oral anticholinergic tablets

- Anti-cholinergic effects are dose-dependent and include dry mouth, blurred vision, constipation, confusion, urinary retention, and tachycardia, amongst others

Treatment pearls

- Topical therapy is considered to be first-line therapy for focal hyperhidrosis given treatment safety and efficacy
- If initial treatment with 12% over-the-counter aluminium chloride fails, prescription 20% aluminium chloride may still be effective
- Aluminum chloride is most effective when applied to dry skin
- Aluminum chloride can be applied under occlusion to increase penetration and efficacy
- Treatment options for irritation associated with aluminium chloride use include reducing the frequency of application and short-term treatment with a topical steroid
- 15% Aluminum chloride in a 2–4% salicylic acid gel (rather than ethanol) may decrease irritation and improve absorption in treatment areas with thicker skin

Further reading

Hoorens I, Ongenae K. Primary focal hyperhidrosis: current treatment options and a step-by-step approach. J Eur Acad Dermatol Venereol 2012; 26:1–8.

Roy K, Forman SB. Miscellaneous topical agents. In: Wolverton SE (ed) Comprehensive Dermatologic Drug Therapy. Philadelphia: Elsevier Health Sciences, 2012. pp. 629–635.

Walling HW, Swick BL. Treatment options for hyperhidrosis. Am J Clin Dermatol 2011; 12:285–295.

Dermatologic indications

- *Licensed indications:* these compounds are available without a prescription

- Chlorhexidine gluconate (CHG) is rapidly bactericidal, with activity against Gram-positive and Gram-negative bacteria as well as some fungi and viruses. It is used in cosmetics, soaps, dental preparations, and surgical scrubs

- Benzalkonium chloride (BAK) is used in cosmetics, eye care products, hair removal products, and topical preparations. It can be used for preoperative disinfection and wound care

- Bleach baths (active ingredient: sodium hypochlorite) are useful against *Staphylococcus aureus* and can be used as adjunctive therapy for decolonization of microbes or recurrent secondarily infected atopic dermatitis as well as in skin and soft tissue infections

- Iodine is rapidly bactericidal with activity against Gram-positive and Gram-negative bacteria as well as *Mycobacterium tuberculosis*, fungi and viruses

- Acetic acid (AA) has activity against staphylococcal and streptococcal species, including MRSA, and Gram-negative organisms. It is most commonly used as a treatment for burn wounds

- Hydrogen peroxide is a general disinfectant with antibacterial and antifungal properties

Background

CHG links to the stratum corneum and remains active, leading to a persistent antimicrobial effect.

Iodine preparations contain free iodine complexed with a surfactant or water-soluble polymer (povidone–iodine [PI]) and combine antiseptic treatment with a favored moist wound environment.

Dermatologic prescribing

- *Chlorhexidine preparations:* concentrations differ depending on the compound used. Chlorhexidine gluconate (CHG) is the most widely available. For the skin, use 2–4% as a wash-off antiseptic/cleanser. Dental preparations to treat periodontitis are commonly 0.12%, and 0.05% is used for wound cleansing and disinfection

- *Preparations containing octenidine:* an alternative for those who suffer an irritant reaction to chlorhexidine

- *Bleach baths (sodium hypochlorite):* to a full bathtub (approximately 120 L), stir in 120 mL

Instructions for bleach baths

Skin may benefit from swimming in pool water due to its antiseptic effects. These instructions make an antiseptic bath at home with a similar concentration to a chlorinated swimming pool

1. Add lukewarm water to fill the bath completely (about 120 L of water)

2. Add 250 mL of 2% sodium hypochlorite sterilizing fluid (e.g. Milton) using a kitchen measuring jug. The amount of sterilizing fluid added may need to be adjusted, depending on the size of the bath and amount of water used

3. Stir the mixture with the jug to make sure the bleach is completely diluted in the bath water

4. The patient should soak in the chlorinated water for 5–10 min

5. Thoroughly rinse skin with lukewarm fresh water at the end of the bleach bath to prevent dryness and irritation

6. As soon as the bath is over, pat the patient dry. Do not rub dry as this is the same as scratching

7. Immediately apply any prescribed medications/emollients

8. Repeat bleach baths twice weekly, or as prescribed

Cautions

- Do not use undiluted bleach directly on the skin. Even diluted bleach can potentially cause dryness and irritation

- Do not use bleach baths if there are many breaks or open areas on the skin (may sting and burn)

- Do not use bleach baths with a known contact allergy to chlorine

of 6% sodium hypochlorite (bleach) or adjust accordingly. Soak for 5–10 minutes, then rinse with fresh water and dry the skin gently. Use twice weekly

- *Benzalkonium chloride (BAK):* available as a 6% antiseptic bath emollient in Europe. A 1:750 concentration is used for preoperative skin preparation

- *Iodine:* povidone–iodine (PI) is available in 5%, 7.5% and 10% formulations. Iodine topical tincture is available as a 2% solution. Numerous wound care products impregnated with iodine are available and are typically applied to clean wounds three times weekly

- *Acetic acid (AA):* concentrations of 0.5–5% are effective in eliminating *Pseudomonas aeruginosa* from superficial infection sites. Of note, vinegar is 5% acetic acid

- *Hydrogen peroxide (HP):* available as a 3% solution
- *Emollients containing chlorhexidine with or without benzalkonium chloride:* are used in secondarily infected atopic dermatitis

Cautions

- No human studies have shown the use of CHG, BAK, AA, or HP on the skin to be harmful in pregnancy. Caution should be exercised in large areas of inflammation, wounds, or burns in case of systemic absorption
- CHG may be ototoxic if it enters the middle ear and can also cause keratitis. CHG is not recommended for infants less than 2 months old
- BAK is an irritant to the middle ear and is associated with drug-induced rhinitis in some studies
- Bleach ingestion or inhalation is associated with significant morbidity and even mortality
- Iodine is toxic if ingested. In high concentration (5%), PI is inhibitory to fibroblasts and may cause adverse effects on wound healing. Although rare, excess use can induce hypothyroidism. PI is contraindicated in burn patients with > 20% body surface area of involvement, newborns, and patients with hypersensitivity to iodides. Use caution in renal failure. Iodine crosses the placenta and is not recommended in pregnancy
- AA in concentrations > 5% can be irritating to the skin
- HP is toxic to fibroblasts and may interfere with wound healing. Do not instill hydrogen peroxide into closed body cavities or abscesses

Common problems

- CHG, BAK and PI can cause irritant contact dermatitis, especially 10% PI solution
- AA can cause skin irritation, headache, nausea, and nasopharyngitis
- Allergic contact dermatitis to CHG, BAK, PI, and sodium hypochlorite should be considered if the skin develops erythema and/or pruritus (although irritant reactions are more common). Rare cases of CHG anaphylaxis have been reported

Treatment pearls

- Topical antiseptic use should be limited to short-term treatment of wound infections in order to avoid interference with wound healing and skin irritation
- Recent studies show preoperative preparation of skin with chlorhexidine is superior to PI for preventing surgical-site infection
- Dilute sodium hypochlorite (bleach) solution has been shown to be an effective adjunctive treatment of staphylococcal colonization and atopic dermatitis
- Cadexomer iodine (e.g. Iodosorb) promotes absorption of fluid, exudate, debris and bacteria from the wound bed, with simultaneous controlled release of iodine at levels that are non-toxic
- AA 3% is a non-toxic, non-irritating and cost-effective treatment strategy for burn wounds and nosocomial infections due to Gram-negative bacteria such as *Proteus vulgaris*, *Acinetobacter baumannii* or *Pseudomonas aeruginosa*
- In addition to AA, aluminum acetate combinations (e.g. Domeboro) are often used in the form of soaks to colonized or infected skin sites as well as to treat otitis externa

Further reading

Darouiche RO, Wall MJ, Itani KMF, et al. Chlorhexidine–alcohol versus povidone–iodine for surgical-site antisepsis. N Engl J Med 2010; 362:18–26.

Huang JT, Abrams M, Tlougan B, et al. Treatment of *Staphylococcus aureus* colonization in atopic dermatitis decreases disease severity. Pediatrics 2009; 123:e808–814.

Kara A, Tezer H, Devrim I, et al. Chemical burn: a risk with outdated povidone iodine. Pediatr Dermatol 2007; 24:449–450.

O'Toole EA, Goel M, Woodley DT. Hydrogen peroxide inhibits human keratinocyte migration. Dermatol Surg 1996; 22:525–529.

Ryssel H, Kloeters O, Germann G, et al. The antimicrobial effect of acetic acid – an alternative to common local antiseptics? Burns 2009; 35:695–700.

Antivirals: acyclovir and penciclovir

Dermatologic indications

- Herpes simplex infection of the skin including lips and genital area, both primary and recurrent infections

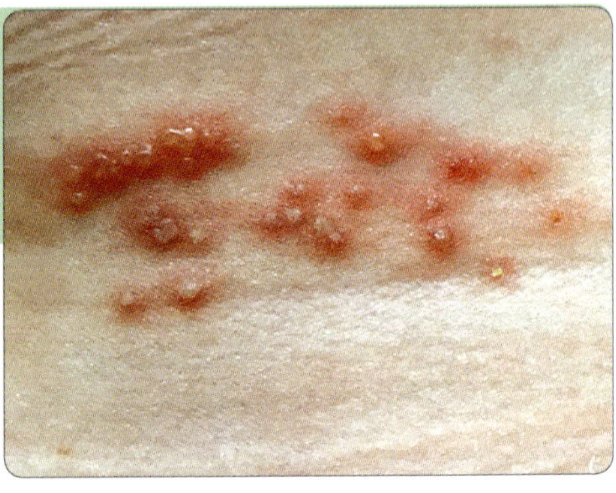

Figure 7.1 Umbilicated vesicles of herpes simplex.

Background

Acyclovir is taken up by mammalian cells and metabolized by a combination of viral and cellular thymidine kinase to acyclovir triphosphate, which can then be incorporated into replicating DNA, halting further DNA production. Penciclovir acts in a similar manner. This chain-terminating effect occurs only in herpes-infected cells, and the drugs have undetectable effects in normal cells.

Acyclovir is active against herpes simplex virus (HSV) 1 and HSV-2, is less effective against varicella zoster virus, and has very limited use in other herpes virus infections such as EBV and CMV.

Primary herpes infection is usually subclinical but can present as a painful gingivostomatitis with erosions around the lips and in the mouth.

Reactivation episodes of herpes labialis may be preceded by symptoms of burning in a localized area, followed within a few hours by the appearance of small erythematous macules or papules. These rapidly develop into fragile vesicles (blisters) which break and evolve into crusted erosions. Healing occurs after a few days but frequently leaves short-lived post-inflammatory pigmentation.

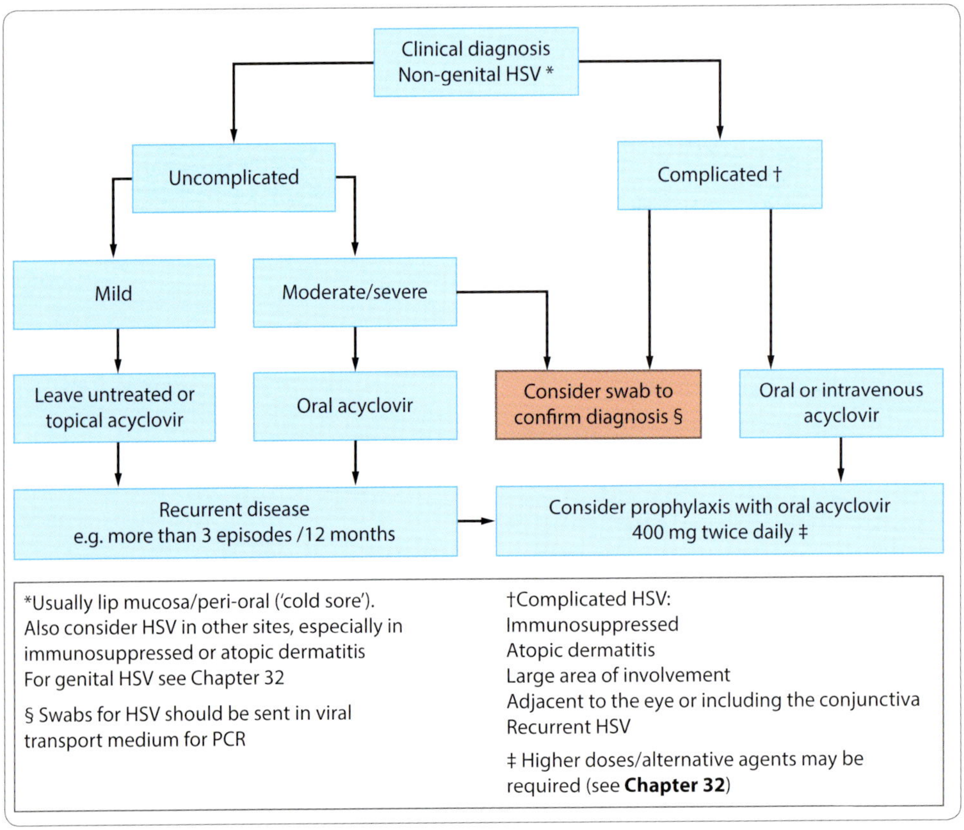

```
                    ┌─────────────────────┐
                    │  Clinical diagnosis  │
                    │  Non-genital HSV *   │
                    └─────────────────────┘
              ┌──────────────┴───────────────┐
      ┌───────────────┐              ┌───────────────┐
      │ Uncomplicated │              │ Complicated † │
      └───────────────┘              └───────────────┘
      ┌───────┴────────┐                     │
  ┌────────┐   ┌───────────────┐             │
  │  Mild  │   │ Moderate/severe│            │
  └────────┘   └───────────────┘             │
      │               │                      │
┌───────────────┐ ┌──────────────┐ ┌──────────────────┐ ┌──────────────────┐
│ Leave untreated│ │Oral acyclovir│ │ Consider swab to │ │Oral or intravenous│
│  or topical    │ │              │ │confirm diagnosis §│ │    acyclovir     │
│   acyclovir    │ │              │ │                  │ │                  │
└───────────────┘ └──────────────┘ └──────────────────┘ └──────────────────┘
      │               │                                          │
┌──────────────────────────────┐   ┌────────────────────────────────────┐
│     Recurrent disease         │   │ Consider prophylaxis with oral      │
│ e.g. more than 3 episodes      │──▶│ acyclovir 400 mg twice daily ‡     │
│       /12 months               │   │                                    │
└──────────────────────────────┘   └────────────────────────────────────┘
```

*Usually lip mucosa/peri-oral ('cold sore'). Also consider HSV in other sites, especially in immunosuppressed or atopic dermatitis
For genital HSV see Chapter 32

§ Swabs for HSV should be sent in viral transport medium for PCR

†Complicated HSV:
Immunosuppressed
Atopic dermatitis
Large area of involvement
Adjacent to the eye or including the conjunctiva
Recurrent HSV

‡ Higher doses/alternative agents may be required (see **Chapter 32**)

Figure 7.2 Treatment algorithm for suspected *Herpes simplex* virus infections e.g. herpes labialis (cold sore).

Reactivation may be triggered by ultraviolet exposure, systemic viral infection, physical trauma at the site, and immunosuppression.

Herpes labialis is usually caused by HSV-1 and less frequently by HSV-2.

Dermatologic prescribing

- 5% acyclovir cream is applied five times daily or every 4 hours to the affected area for 5–10 days

- 1% penciclovir cream is used every 2 hours during waking hours, i.e. 8 times daily for 4 days

- Moderate/severe infections: oral or intravenous treatment (see **Chapter 32**)

Cautions

- Avoid if known allergic to acyclovir, famciclovir, valacyclovir, or components of the base such as propylene glycol or cetosteryl alcohol

- No problems have been recorded in pregnancy or breast feeding

- Topical acyclovir is not recommended for use in genital herpes or for primary infection

Common problems

- The penetration of acyclovir through intact epidermis is poor, making the treatment window limited

- The frequency of application (5 times daily for acyclovir and 8 times daily for penciclovir) can make compliance difficult

- Acyclovir and penciclovir creams are irritants to mucosal surfaces. Contact with the eye, oral cavity, or genital mucosa should be avoided

- Studies of topical acyclovir have not shown convincing evidence of pain reduction, but duration of lesions may be reduced by 0.5–2 days

- There is no convincing evidence that topical acyclovir has an effect when used prophylactically before UV exposure

Treatment pearls

- Treatment should be started as soon as possible, even before lesions appear. Patients should be instructed to start application at the time of prodrome (typically burning or stinging at the site). If the disease worsens despite 2 days of treatment, consider switching to oral therapy

- Clinical impressions suggest that more frequent application, such as hourly, may improve efficacy, but this has not been formally demonstrated in a study, and irritant dermatitis is a frequent limiting complication

- Penciclovir 1% cream may offer a slight benefit in terms of decreasing the duration of pain and time to healing compared to 5% acyclovir cream. Penciclovir cream has not been tested in children and is not licenced for use in children under 12 years of age

- If reactivation episodes are frequent, oral acyclovir can be considered

- If the patient is immunosuppressed oral anti-viral therapy should be used, both to improve efficacy and to avoid the risk of selection of acyclovir-resistant strains

- Acyclovir cream has a 3-year shelf life in a cool room (not refrigerated)

Further reading

Boon R, Goodman JJ, Martinez J, et al. Penciclovir cream for the treatment of sunlight-induced herpes simplex labialis: a randomized, double-blind, placebo-controlled trial. Penciclovir Cream Herpes Labialis Study Group. Clin Ther 2000; 22:76–90.

Cunningham A, Griffiths P, Leone P, et al. Current management and recommendations for access to antiviral therapy of herpes labialis. J Clin Virol 2012; 53:6–11.

Hull CM, Harmenberg J, Arlander E, et al. Early treatment of cold sores with topical ME-609 decreases the frequency of ulcerative lesions: A randomized, double-blind, placebo-controlled, patient-initiated clinical trial. J Am Acad Dermatol 2011; 64:696.e1–696.e11.

Rahimi H, Mara T, Costella J, et al. Effectiveness of antiviral agents for the prevention of recurrent herpes labialis: a systematic review and meta-analysis. Oral Surg Oral Med Oral Pathol Oral Radiol 2012; 113:618–627.

Calcineurin inhibitors

Dermatologic indications

- Atopic dermatitis
- *Widely used for:* vitiligo, lichen planus, lichen sclerosus, psoriasis (especially genital and facial)
- *Also used for:* cutaneous lupus erythematosus, dermatomyositis, morphea, periorificial dermatitis, chronic graft-versus-host disease, seborrheic dermatitis, rosacea

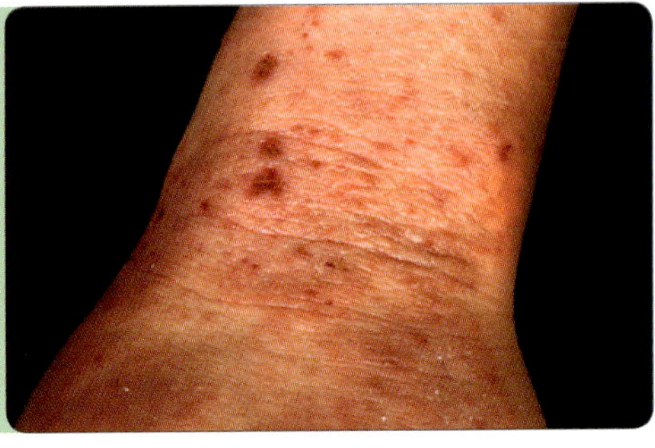

Figure 8.1 Chronic lichenified atopic dermatitis on the wrist flexure. Calcineurin inhibitors are ideally suited for skin where the risk of cutaneous atrophy with prolonged use of topical corticosteroids is greatest, such as the face and flexures.

Background

Topical calcineurin inhibitors (TCI) are anti-inflammatory agents that inhibit the production of pro-inflammatory cytokines.

Antigen binding to T-cell receptors increases intracellular calcium, which binds to and activates calmodulin and subsequently calcineurin. Calcineurin dephosphorylates nuclear factor of activated T-cells (NFAT). NFAT is subsequently translocated to the nucleus where it assists in cytokine transcription. Inhibition of calcineurin results in decreased cytokine transcription and reduced T-cell activity.

Tacrolimus and pimecrolimus are used as topical corticosteroid-sparing agents to prevent side effects from topical corticosteroids such as cutaneous atrophy, telangiectasias, striae, perioral dermatitis, cataracts, and glaucoma.

TCI use as maintenance therapy has demonstrated a reduced number of flares and an increase time to flare in atopic dermatitis.

Dermatologic prescribing

- Topical application is typically twice daily during times of disease activity
- Topical application is typically twice daily for 2 days per week for maintenance therapy
- Application to acutely inflamed skin is not recommended as this will often cause stinging and discomfort
- Utilized as a topical corticosteroid-sparing agent, particularly in areas of thin skin (face, eyelids, skin folds, and genitals) where chronic topical corticosteroid use is more likely to result in atrophy
- Tacrolimus is manufactured as 0.1% and 0.03% ointment. Pimecrolimus is manufactured as 1% cream. Both pimecrolimus and tacrolimus in 0.03% formulation are approved for children 2 years of age or older. Tacrolimus in 0.1% formulation is approved for patients aged 15 years or older.

Cautions

- *Black box warning:* in 2005, the FDA released a warning regarding a theoretical risk of Hodgkin's and non-Hodgkin's lymphoma, melanoma, and non-melanoma skin cancers with chronic TCI use. This theoretical risk assessment was based on in vitro studies and systemic and dermal administration in animal studies. Short and intermediate (>10 year) post-marketing surveillance has demonstrated no increased risk of malignancy; in fact, fewer cases of malignancy were reported in patients treated with TCI compared to that expected for the general population
- *Sun:* Most dermatologists advise patients using TCIs to avoid prolonged sun exposure on the treated skin, especially in conditions with a high UV index (>6). If unavoidable, then high factor sunscreens should be applied or a switch to topical corticosteroids recommended. This advice is likely to be less of a concern in those with low background risk of skin cancer (e.g. dark skin).
- *Infection:* numerous studies show a trend (not statistically significant) toward an increase in viral skin infections (HSV, VZV, HPV) in patients treated with TCI. In contrast, *Staphylococcus aureus* colonization is decreased in AD patients treated with TCI
- *Systemic absorption:* detectable, albeit low, serum levels have been measured after topical tacrolimus and pimecrolimus application

in infants, children, and adults. However, these low serum levels have not resulted in immune suppression. TCIs have not been approved for children less than 2 years of age due to a higher surface area per weight ratio. Patients with Netherton syndrome and lamellar ichthyosis have an abnormal epidermis and may develop substantial plasma levels of tacrolimus when applied topically; therefore, TCI use in these patients is relatively contraindicated

- *Medication interactions:* no known medication interactions

- *Pregnancy/lactation risk:* No adequate studies have been performed. TCIs are secreted in breast milk and are not recommended during breast feeding

Common problems

- Site reactions including burning and stinging

- Erythema, irritation, and pruritus are also reported side effects

- Concurrent alcohol consumption may cause flushing

Further reading

Callen J, Chamlin S, Eichenfield C, et al. A systematic review of the safety of topical therapies for atopic dermatitis. Br J Dermatol 2007; 156:203–221.

Siegfried EC, Jaworski JC, Hebert AA. Topical calcineurin inhibitors and lymphoma risk: Evidence update with implications for daily practice. Am J Clin Dermatol 2013; 14:163–178.

Thaci D, Reitamo S, Gonzalez-Ensenat MA, et al. Proactive disease management with 0.03% tacrolimus ointment for children with atopic dermatitis: results of a randomized, multicenter, comparative study. Br J Dermatol 2008; 159:1348–1356.

Treatment pearls

- TCIs are commonly used as part of a maintenance therapy plan with the goal of decreasing flares. Local site reactions from TCIs are more common in flaring skin. Therefore, if patients have a severe flare of their dermatitis, reversion to topical corticosteroids for 1–2 weeks is recommended for flare management

- A common maintenance regimen is 2 days per week of twice daily TCI application

- For patients with frequent AD flares, a common maintenance regimen is 5 days per week of twice daily TCI and 2 days per week of topical corticosteroid ointment as needed

- If burning or stinging occur upon application, the medication can be stored in the refrigerator, which has anecdotally been reported to decrease these sensations

Corticosteroids

Dermatologic indications

- *Common dermatologic indications:* atopic dermatitis (atopic eczema), allergic and irritant contact dermatitis
- *Also used for:* other inflammatory skin conditions including seborrheic dermatitis, psoriasis, lichen planus, cutaneous lupus erythematosus, alopecia areata, hypertrophic scarring, lichen sclerosus et atrophicus, insect bite reactions, bullous pemphigoid and hypersensitivity reactions

Background

Less accurately called 'topical steroids', these agents are agonists of the glucocorticoid receptor, which regulates gene transcription, resulting in a wide range of anti-inflammatory and immunosuppressant effects.

Infants and young children are particularly prone to topical steroid-induced side effects, but the risk is minimized by using an appropriate strength corticosteroid for an appropriate duration.

Corticosteroids suppress inflammation, but 'rebound' may occur after discontinuation of treatment.

Dermatologic prescribing

- Corticosteroids can be applied to the skin in ointments (oil-based formulations), creams and lotions (water-based formulations), sprays or steroid-impregnated adhesive tape

- Four groups of topical corticosteroids exist according to potency: mild, moderate, potent, and very potent

- The UK classification uses four steps while clinicians in the US use seven classes:

  - *Very potent (Class I):* e.g. clobetasol propionate

  - *Potent (Class II):* e.g. mometasone furoate, betamethasone dipropionate

  - *Moderate (Class III–IV):* e.g. clobetasone butyrate, triamcinolone acetonide 0.1%

  - *Mild (Class V–VII):* e.g. hydrocortisone

- Classification is based on the 'vasoconstrictor assay', which compares induction of vasoconstriction in the skin of healthy volunteers by the topical agent

  - This does not always precisely reflect the relative efficacy in treating an inflammatory skin disease

- Ointments are more effective, because they have a greater moisturising action, which promotes

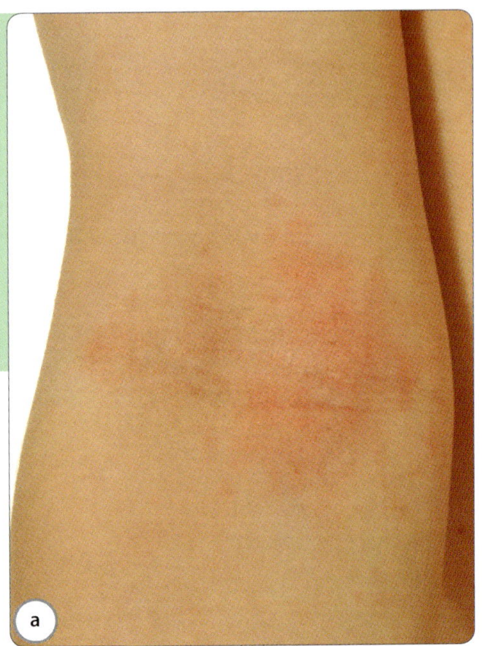

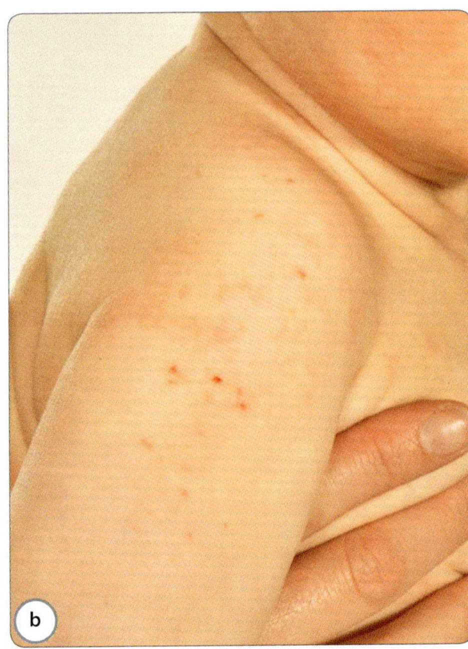

Figure 9.1 Two common indications for corticosteroids.
(a) Atopic dermatitis (synonymous with atopic eczema) showing typical flexural involvement.
(b) Diffuse atopic dermatitis on the trunk and upper limb with excoriations.
(Courtesy of Department of Medical Photography, Ninewells Hospital and Medical School, Dundee).

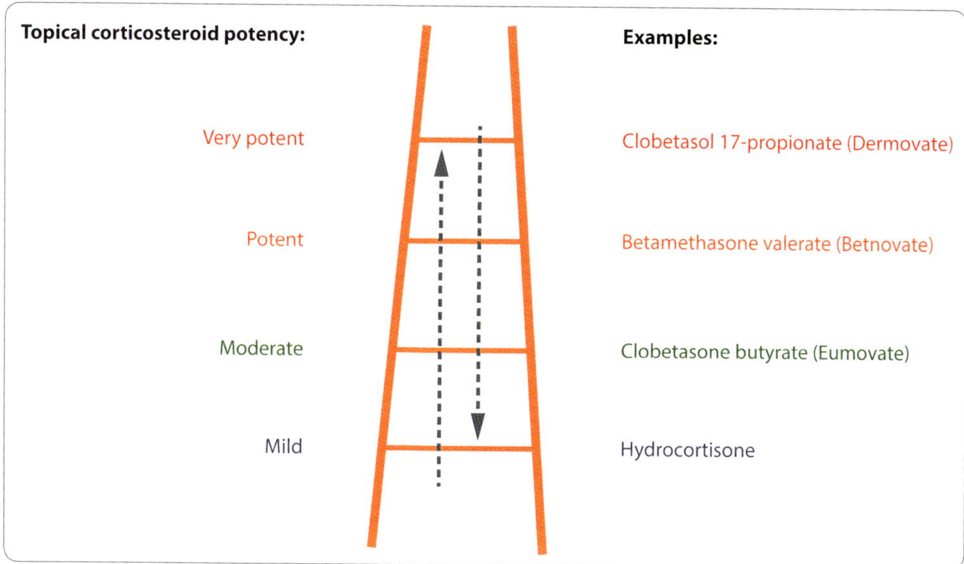

Figure 9.2 Topical corticosteroid 'ladder'.

drug penetration through the stratum corneum. However, they may be disliked due to their greasy nature or 'stickiness'. Ointments are not suitable for exudative areas

- Creams may be preferred for cosmetic reasons. Lotion, gel, mousse, foam, oil or shampoo formulations are preferred for hair bearing skin

- Adhesive tape can be used to apply corticosteroids to a controlled area, such as an area of inflammatory fissuring on fingers or a region of hypertrophic scarring

- Mild and moderately potent formulations are suitable for long-term therapy of chronic eczematous disorders, ensuring the appropriate breaks from therapy to avoid local side effects. They can be used on the face and flexures when required

- Potent and very potent corticosteroids are best used for short periods of up to 4 weeks, for more severe dermatoses, and usually on the trunk, limbs or scalp

- Mild-to-moderate potency topical corticosteroids are not associated with a risk of systemic side effects, in contrast to oral

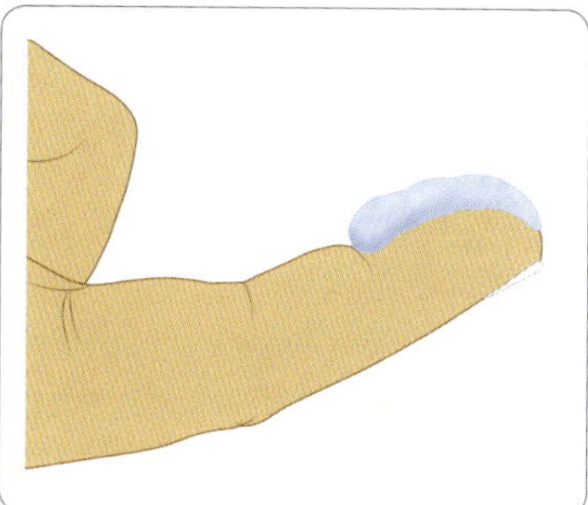

Figure 9.3 A finger tip unit (FTU).

or intravenous routes. Very potent topical corticosteroids (and rarely potent formulations) can induce suppression of the hypothalamic–pituitary–adrenal axis when used on large areas

- Finger tip units:
    - 500 mg is estimated by a line of cream or ointment from the distal finger crease to the end of the finger tip: a finger tip unit, FTU
    - One adult finger tip unit treats an area the size of two adult hand prints

Common problems

- Long-term application of topical corticosteroids (usually potent or very potent corticosteroids applied over many months or years) may induce atrophy of the skin, which manifests as thinning, fragility, dyspigmentation, telangiectasia, and purpura. The most vulnerable sites include the face, groin, flexures or occluded sites

- Atrophy is prevented by using the appropriate strength of topical corticosteroid in the appropriate place for the appropriate duration

- Misplaced fear of topical corticosteroids ('steroid phobia') is relatively common, results in treatment non-adherence, and should be considered as a cause of therapy failure

- On facial skin, and less often at other sites, topical corticosteroids can induce a variety of acneiform reactions including acne vulgaris, rosacea, and perioral or periocular dermatitis. Once present, these reactions may take months to resolve

- 'Tachyphylaxis' has been used to describe a gradual loss of efficacy over months. The mechanism is controversial but may be due to a variety of drug and patient factors

- Adverse effects are mostly confined to the skin. However, central suppression of the hypothalamic–pituitary–adrenal axis is recognized with extensive use. Most risk arises in children or subjects using >50 g of very potent formulations per week

Treatment pearls

- Topical corticosteroids should be applied to areas of active inflammation when skin is fully hydrated (for example, after bathing), to maximize absorption

- Once-daily application has been shown to be as effective as twice-daily application in eczema treatment, with a lower risk of side effects

- When adequate control of the underlying condition is achieved, step down to a less potent topical corticosteroid before withdrawing the treatment, to reduce the risk of relapse

- Using topical corticosteroids as maintenance therapy (e.g. 'weekend treatment': 2 consecutive days/week) on previously active sites may help to reduce flare-ups in moderate severe eczema

- Written treatment plans and a multidisciplinary approach to educate patients and caregivers improves compliance and reduces adverse effects

- Potent topical corticosteroids applied for a few days can be very useful in reducing the dermatitis and pruritus associated with scabies. It is critical that the infestation is treated as well

- Short term corticosteroid-induced vasoconstriction in acne or rosacea may give the false impression of a beneficial effect. The disease will not fully respond and will eventually flare

- Accidental treatment of a dermatophyte (fungus) infection with topical corticosteroids will provide short term improvement in itching and inflammation, but the infection will extend and worsen

- Although topical corticosteroids are often used in contact dermatitis, the primary treatment should be to avoid the allergen or irritant

- Treatment of insect bites and stings may be unsuccessful and typically requires potent topical corticosteroids to observe improvement. Mild preparations available over-the-counter have little evidence of efficacy

- Occlusion of topical corticosteroids with hydrocolloid dressings, polythene gloves, or film (cling film or saran wrap) can markedly increase penetration. This is often useful in refractory hand eczema, lichen simplex chronicus, and hypertrophic inflammatory lesions. Side effects will also be enhanced

- Compound formulations combining corticosteroids with other drugs (e.g. antibiotics or antifungals) should be used only when there is an indication for each of the constituents

Table 9.1 Treatment dosage for acne and rosacea

Area of body	Creams and ointments/2 weeks (adult)
Face and neck	15–30 g
Both hands	15–30 g
Scalp	15–30 g
Both arms	30–60 g
Both legs	100 g
Trunk	100 g
Groin and genitalia	15 to 30 g

- If applying once daily, the above quantities will be enough for 2 weeks use
- Mild potency cortcosteroids are recommended as teh mainstay of treatment in infants and areas of the body where skin absorption is greatest (face, neck, flexures and groin)
- Short-term increases in potency may be appropriate for disease flares
- Caution is required in the regular use of potent or very potent corticosteroids
- Prescriptions for children should be weaker potency and smaller amounts

Further reading

Berth-Jones J, Damstra RJ, Golsch S, et al. Twice weekly fluticasone propionate added to emollient maintenance treatment to reduce risk of relapse in atopic dermatitis: randomised, double blind, parallel-group study. Br Med J 2003; 326:1367–1370.

Bewley A on behalf of the Dermatology Working Group. Expert consensus: time for a change in the way we advise our patients to use topical corticosteroids. Br J Dermatol 2008; 158:917–920.

Eichenfield LF, Tom WL, Berger TG, et al. Guidelines of care for the management of atopic dermatitis: section 2. Management and treatment of atopic dermatitis with topical therapies. J Am Acad Dermatol 2014; 71:116–132.

Tang TS, Bieber T, Williams HC. Are the concepts of induction of remission and treatment of subclinical inflammation in atopic dermatitis clinically useful? J Allergy Clin Immunol 2014; 133:1615–1625.

Williams HC. Established corticosteroid creams should be applied only once daily in patients with atopic eczema. BMJ 2007; 334:1272.

Depigmenting agents

Dermatologic indications

- Hyperpigmentation: often caused by melasma or post-inflammatory changes

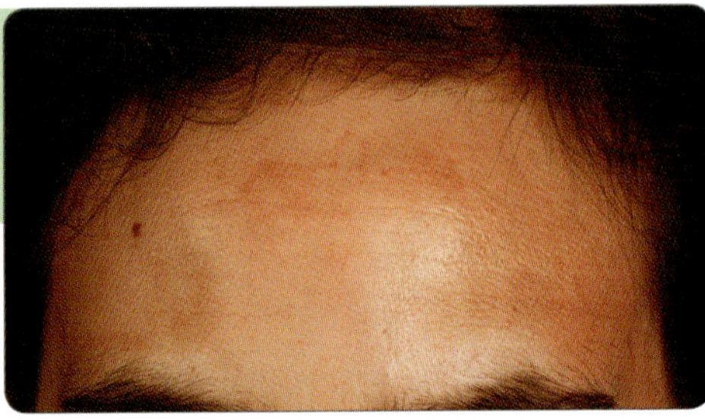

Figure 10.1 Melasma on the forehead.

Background

Inflammation causing melanocyte activation can result in hyperpigmentation. This process occurs more in darker skin and may follow skin trauma including that from atopic dermatitis, burns, acne, infection and lichenoid rashes. This melanocyte activation results in increased melanin deposition in epidermal cells as well as pigment granules in between cells in the dermis. Melanin deep in the epidermis or within intercellular spaces in the dermis is unlikely to be successfully treated topically.

Melasma presents with brown to gray-brown facial pigmentation and involves melanin deposition in the epidermis and dermis. Melasma is associated with pregnancy, hormone therapies, ultraviolet exposure and certain medications.

Drug-induced hyperpigmentation can be caused by NSAIDs, phenytoin, amiodarone, antimalarials, antipsychotics, tetracyclines, cytotoxic drugs and heavy metals. These changes are often due to increased melanin deposition, but can be due to deposition of the drug in the dermis (such as with heavy metals) with formation of a drug-pigment complex, or to the accumulation of a drug in the skin reacting with other substances.

Dermatologic prescribing

- Hydroquinone is a depigmenting agent that has been banned in cosmetics in the EU since 2001

- In the US, products containing up to 2% hydroquinone may be sold without a prescription. Prescription products may contain up to 4% hydroquinone (4% hydroquinone may be prescribed as a monotherapy, e.g. Lustra and EpiQuin Micro which are both 4% hydroquinone cream, or in combination as Triluma (a combination of hydroquinone 4%, fluocinolone acetonide 0.01%, and tretinoin 0.05%)

- Hydroquinone products are readily available for unregulated purchase throughout Europe, Asia, and Africa

- In the UK, there are no licensed depigmenting agents, but topical acne treatments can induce exfoliation and decrease hyperpigmentation. This is thought to be partly due to epidermal peeling, but also to reduction of epidermal melanin production by inhibition of tyrosinase

- Topical application of hydroquinone produces a reversible depigmentation of the skin by inhibition of the enzymatic oxidation of tyrosine to 3,4-dihydroxyphenylalanine as well as suppression of other melanocyte metabolic processes

- Agents used to treat superficial hyperpigmentation include:

  - *Azelaic acid:* Skinoren cream (20% azelaic acid), Finacea gel (15% azelaic acid)

  - *Topical retinoids:* Isotrex gel (0.05% isotretinoin, 0.025%, 0.05%, 0.1% tretinoin gel/cream)

  - *Adapelene:* Differin (0.1% gel/cream)

  - *Hydroquinone:* Pigmanorm (5% hydroquinone, 1% hydrocortisone and 0.1% tretinoin can be obatined in the UK but is prescribed as an off-license medication. Triluma (hydroquinone 4%, fluocinolone acetonide 0.01%, tretinoin 0.05%

- Cosmetics can also contain agents thought to reduce pigmentation such as: fruit acids, ascorbic acid (vitamin C), kojic acid, arbutin (bearberry), licorice, mequinol, niacinamide, *N*-acetyl glucosamine and soy

Common problems

- Irritation
- Incomplete efficacy
- Unwanted hypopigmentation

Less common problems include:

- Ochronosis is an adverse effect associated with long-term hydroquinone use. This blue/black skin discoloration is secondary to deposition of yellow or ochre-colored deposits in the dermis. Similar pigment changes in the skin are seen in patients with alkaptonuria as well as in those exposed to chemicals such as phenol, mercury, picric acid, benzene, and antimalarials. These pigment changes are due to the accumulation of homogentisic acid and should be avoided by limiting use of hydroquinone to no more than 2–3 months

- Hydroquinone may act as a carcinogen although its cancer-causing properties have yet to be proven in humans

- Hydroquinone contains sulfites, which can cause allergic reactions in certain susceptible individuals such as asthmatics

Further reading

Denton CR, Lerner AB, Fitzpatrick TB. Inhibition of melanin formation by chemical agents. J Invest Dermatol 1952 18:119–135.

Dogra S, Kanwar AJ, Parsad D. Adapalene in the treatment of melasma: a preliminary report. J Dermatol 2002; 29:539–540.

Jimbow K, Obata M, Pathak MA, Fitzpatrick TB. Mechanisms of depigmentation by hydroquinone. J Invest Dermatol 1974; 62:436–449.

Rivas S, Pandya AG. Treatment of melasma with topical agents, peels and lasers: and evidence based review. Am J Clin Dermatol 2013; 14:359-76.

Sofen B, Prado G, Emer J. Melasma and post inflammatory hyperpigmentation: management update and expert opinion. Skin Therapy Lett 2016; 21:1-7.

Treatment pearls

- Erythema and skin peeling can occur with topical depigmenting treatments. Exposure time can be reduced in these cases by washing creams off after a short period of time, such as 4 hours, and gradually increasing thereafter

- Excessive irritation should be avoided as this in itself may lead to post-inflammatory hyperpigmentation in susceptible individuals

- Up to 6 months of treatment may be required to see beneficial effects with topical treatments (hydroquinone use should be limited to 2–3 months)

- Diligent photoprotection with sunscreen and the use of a wide-brimmed hat is an essential component of therapy to reduce pigmentation as any ultraviolet exposure sustains melanocytic activity and can worsen hyperpigmentation or re-pigment treated areas

- Hydroquinone cream should not be used with products that contain hydrogen peroxide or benzoyl peroxide as this may cause a dark staining of the skin. This staining, however, may be removed by washing the skin with soap and water

Depilatory treatments

Depilatory treatments

Dermatologic indications

- Topical eflornithine is licensed for facial hirsutism in women over 18 years of age
- Other treatments used to reduce unwanted hair include oral contraceptive pills, anti-androgen systemic therapy, electrolysis, intense pulsed light and laser hair removal

Background

- The degree of unwanted body hair varies in severity, and the desire for hair removal varies among cultures
- Hirsutism is abnormal terminal hair growth in women in androgen-dependent sites
- Hypertrichosis is excess hair growth at non-androgen dependent sites
- Excessive hair can be caused by an endocrine abnormality, a medication, or a paraneoplastic syndrome. It is critical to evaluate for possible underlying causes prior to treatment

Dermatologic prescribing

- Eflornithine 13.9% cream
  - Inhibits ornithine decarboxylase, arresting follicular matrix cell proliferation
  - Apply topically twice daily to affected areas for up to 24 weeks. May cause burning or an acneiform eruption. Studies of its use in pregnancy or nursing are lacking
  - May cause burning or an acneiform eruption
- Oral contraceptive pills (OCPs) may be effective in the treatment of hirsutism
  - Choose OCPs with combined estrogen with either low or anti-androgen progestin
  - OCPs suppress ovarian androgen synthesis and decrease free testosterone by increasing sex hormone binding globulin
  - Contraindicated in smokers (>35 years old), patients with a history of cardiovascular disease, uncontrolled hypertension, thromboembolic disorders, breast cancer, and if pregnancy is suspected. OCPs increase the risk of venous thromboembolism
- Anti-androgen systemic therapy for moderate-to-severe hirsutism (see **Chapter 25**)
  - Inhibits androgen receptor and reduces 5α-reductase enzyme activity
  - Spironolactone 50–200 mg daily is the first-line treatment
  - Contraindications include pregnancy, breastfeeding
  - Adverse effects include hyperkalemia, hypotension, breast tenderness, menstrual irregularities, teratogenic, and rarely, hepatotoxicity

Non-permanent physical hair removal

- Plucking, shaving, waxing, bleaching, chemical depilatories

Permanent or long-lasting hair removal

Electrolysis

- Electrical current delivered by fine needle destroys follicle
- Requires multiple treatments, tedious, and efficacy is operator-dependent
- Option for patients who are not good candidates for laser hair removal (e.g. light hairs, fine hairs)

Intense pulsed light (IPL) or laser hair removal

- This is the most-requested cosmetic procedure worldwide
- Hair follicles are targeted using the theory of selective photothermolysis. Energy is delivered to the skin at a wavelength that is absorbed by melanin located primarily in the hair shaft, converted to heat that diffuses and damages stem cells in the bulge region
- Patient selection is important as the best results occur with non-pigmented or light skin types and dark hair. Treatment of darker skin types can result in energy being absorbed by the normal skin, causing burning and/or dyspigmentation. Pale hairs do not absorb the energy and are unaffected
- The aim is long-term significant reduction rather than permanent, complete hair removal. Multiple treatments are required and it is important to counsel patients regarding expectations
- A history of recurrent herpes simplex virus (HSV) infection at the treatment site may warrant antiviral prophylaxis

- A history of keloids or hypertrophic scarring may require more conservative therapy
- Caution should be observed in patients with a history of gold exposure, given the risk of chrysiasis
- Waiting 6–12 months after isotretinoin therapy prior to laser treatment is advised
- Waiting 2–6 weeks after hair removal methods that target the hair shaft (e.g. waxing) is necessary
- Treating the periorbital area and glabella should be avoided, due to the risk of eye injury
- There is an increased risk of adverse events in patients with darker skin types as epidermal melanin competes with the hair follicle target. Consider using a longer wavelength laser, such as the Nd:YAG (1064 nm), as there is less epidermal melanin absorption
- If a tan is present, delay treatment or adjust the laser parameters accordingly

Common problems

- Treatments do not typically result in full hair removal
- The most common side effects of laser hair removal are pain, transient erythema, and perifollicular edema; severe side effects include hyperpigmentation or hypopigmentation, blisters, burns, or scarring. Ocular damage, HSV reactivation and chrysiasis may also occur

Further reading

Gan SD, Graber EM. Laser hair removal: a review. Dermatol Surg 2013; 39:823–838.

Ibrahimi OA, Avram MM, Hanke CW, et al. Laser hair removal. Dermatol Ther 2011; 24:94–107.

Somani N, Turvy D. Hirsutism: an evidence-based treatment update. Am J Clin Dermatol 2014; 15:247–266.

Treatment pearls

- Topical anesthesia for laser hair removal may be applied 30 minutes to 1 hour before treatment. The treatment area should be limited in size because of rare reports of lidocaine toxicity or methemoglobinemia (with prilocaine)
- Everyone in the treatment room, patient and operator, must wear wavelength-specific eye protection during laser treatment
- Laser device parameter selection is crucial for treatment efficacy and to avoid complications. Variables differ between devices
- The optimal laser fluence will produce the clinical endpoint of perifollicular erythema and edema. Higher fluence will lead to greater hair reduction, but can produce excessive heat and consequent side effects
- After a laser hair removal procedure, cooled air or ice-packs should be applied to the treated areas. Topical corticosteroids may also be applied. Strict sun avoidance and sun protection are needed for at least 6 weeks after treatment
- Erythema and edema are expected for 2 days following laser hair removal, but may be present for up to 1 week after treatment

Dithranol

Dermatologic indications

- Psoriasis (plaque)
- *Also used for:* alopecia areata (unlicensed)

Background

Dithranol (also known as anthralin) is a synthetically produced analogue of chrysarobin, an extract from the South American araroba tree, which was historically used for the treatment of skin diseases, including psoriasis.

The precise mechanism of action remains unclear, although dithranol is known to localize to mitochondria and target the respiratory chain, resulting in apoptosis (programmed cell death). Dithranol may also inhibit cell proliferation, which is characteristic of psoriasis.

According to the UK National Institute for Health and Care Excellence (NICE) guidelines, 'short contact dithranol' (see below) should be considered for psoriasis affecting the limbs and trunk that has been resistant to first line treatment (topical corticosteroids and vitamin D analogs).

Dermatologic prescribing

- Proprietary preparations of dithranol are available at concentrations between 0.1–5%. These are most suited for home use and are usually washed off after 5–60 minutes, which is known as 'short contact dithranol'. Dithranol is available as an ointment, a cream and a scalp gel

- Treatments are repeated once or twice daily until clearance is achieved

- Treatment should be commenced with a low concentration of dithranol e.g. 0.1% and gradually increased to the maximum concentration tolerated, every few days

- Typically, 6–12 weeks of treatment are needed to achieve clearance

- In some countries, nurse specialists may apply intensive treatments, either as an inpatient or outpatient, with dithranol pastes or ointments under dressings that are left on for longer periods (usually overnight or throughout the day)

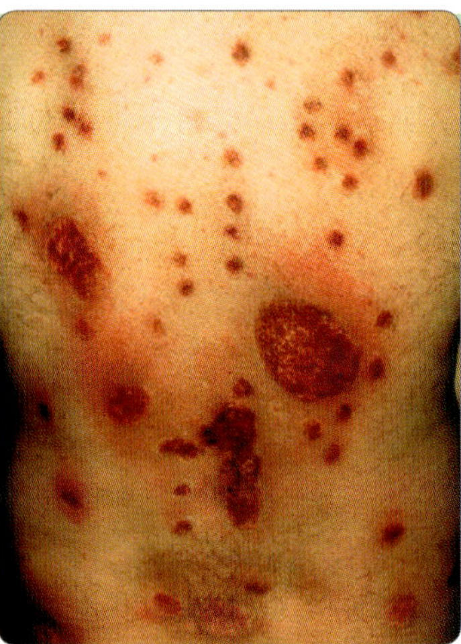

Figure 12.1 Dithranol staining of the skin. This is harmless and will gradually disappear following discontinuation of treatment.

Cautions

- Treatment should be applied to psoriatic plaques only: application to normal skin or broken skin should be avoided

- Use should also be avoided in inflammatory or pustular psoriasis, near the eyes, or in flexural areas, as this frequently results in irritation

- Application to the face should only be undertaken with specialist supervision, due to sensitivity and skin staining

- Use should be discontinued if acute inflammation occurs as continued use may result in unstable psoriasis

Common problems

- Dithranol stains skin and hair brown or purple. This is harmless and will gradually disappear after discontinuation of treatment. The skin should not be scrubbed, as this will worsen the psoriasis. Staining of hair will grow out

- Dithranol also stains fabrics, sometimes permanently

- Irritation and burning of normal skin adjacent to psoriasis plaques may occur

Treatment pearls

- Treatment should commence with a low concentration (0.1%) of dithranol. If there is no improvement and no evidence of irritation after 7–10 days, the strength can be increased, typically to 0.25%. Subsequent increases in dithranol concentration can be made every few days (to a maximum concentration of 2%)

- After the desired contact time (beginning initially with 5 minutes, before increasing after a few days up to 60 minutes if no irritation occurs), dithranol should be removed with cotton wool soaked in oil or a mild detergent. The patient should then shower or bathe

- The maximum achievable concentration and duration of dithranol contact will depend on individual patient tolerability

- If irritation occurs, either the duration of contact, the frequency of application, or the concentration should be reduced. Application should be discontinued if severe inflammation occurs

- For treatment of the scalp, the hair should be parted and dithranol rubbed into the affected areas. The patient should then shampoo the medication off after about 30 minutes. Dithranol may be unsuitable for patients with light hair due to staining

- When applying dithranol, gloves should be worn, or hands washed afterwards

- To avoid staining of the bath/shower, residual dithranol should be washed off immediately with hot water and suitable cleaner or bleach

- Patient adherence with topical treatments can be particularly problematic, with studies showing non-adherence rates of up to 39%, with up to 95% of patients under-dosing their topical treatments. To aid with adherence, patients may benefit from demonstrations, regular follow-up, and membership of a support group (e.g. The Psoriasis Association). Patients with dexterity issues may benefit from additional support

- If the patient is using other topical medications (e.g. emollients), they should be applied at a different time of day or after washing off dithranol

- Dithranol is not suitable for widespread small lesions

- Dithranol is not effective in the treatment of nail psoriasis

Further reading

McBride SR, Walker P, Reynolds NJ. Optimising the frequency of outpatient short contact dithranol treatment: a randomised, within patient controlled trial. Br J Dermatol 2003; 149:1259–1265.

McGill A, Frank A, Emmett N, et al. The anti-psoriatic drug anthralin accumulates in keratinocyte mitochondria, dissipates mitochondrial membrane potential, and induces apoptosis through a pathway dependent on respiratory competent mitochondria. FASEB Journal 2005;19:1012–1014.

National Institute for Health and Care Excellence. NICE guidelines CG153. Psoriasis: Assessment and management of psoriasis. London: NICE, 2012.

Runne U, Kunze J. Short-duration ('minutes') therapy with dithranol for psoriasis: a new out-patient regimen. Br J Dermatol 1982; 106:135–139.

Emollients

Dermatologic indications

- Dry and scaling skin conditions (i.e. xerosis and ichthyosis)
- Inflammatory dermatoses, e.g. eczema and psoriasis
- Widely used as: soap substitutes and bath additives

Background

Emollients hydrate and help to soften the epidermis. They also provide a weak physical barrier, protecting the skin from external environmental factors and helping to reduce water loss.

Regular emollient application is first-line treatment for mild eczema (atopic dermatitis); emollients are used in combination with topical corticosteroids in moderate-severe eczema and other inflammatory skin conditions (see **Chapter 9**).

Emollients are available both as 'leave-on' preparations (ointments, creams, lotions, and sprays) and 'wash-off' products.

Dermatologic prescribing

- Adults require 250–500 g per week, or >1 kg/week for widespread eczema or ichthyosis
- Ointments are oil-based; creams and lotions are water-based emollients
- The choice of preparation depends on patient preference and practicality for their daily activities

Ointments

- These are generally the most effective emollients, but cannot be used on skin that is wet, on skin that is weeping or oozing; some patients also dislike the 'greasy' sensation
- *Non-proprietary examples include:* liquid paraffin and white soft paraffin (50% each); emulsifying ointment (emulsifying wax 30%, white soft paraffin 50%, liquid paraffin 20%)
- *Proprietary examples include:* Epaderm ointment and Hydromol ointment (each yellow soft paraffin 30%, liquid paraffin 40%, emulsifying wax 30%)

Creams and gels

- Creams and gels are easier to apply and patients may find them more cosmetically acceptable than ointments
- *Proprietary examples include:* Oilatum (light liquid paraffin 6%, white soft paraffin 15%); Doublebase gel (liquid paraffin 15%, isopropyl myristate 15%)

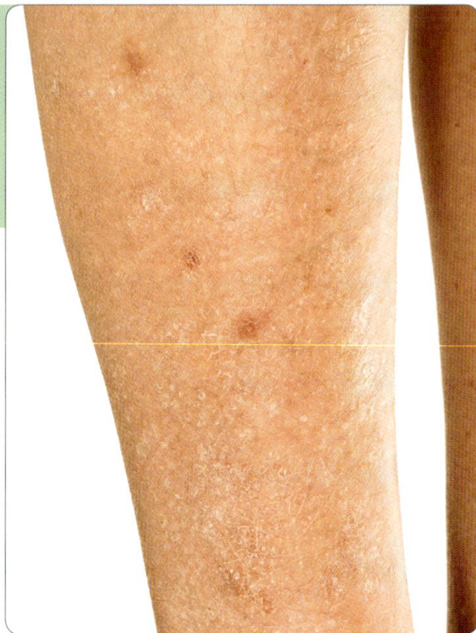

Figure 13.1 Xerosis and mild ichthyosis on the legs of an elderly patient. Courtesy of Department of Medical Photography, Ninewells Hospital and Medical School, Dundee.

Lotions

- Lotions are water-based and lighter than creams, and are therefore suitable for hair-bearing skin
- *Proprietary examples include:* QV lotion (white soft paraffin 5%); Aveeno lotion (colloidal oatmeal)

Sprays

- Oil-based emollients which can be applied quickly in a thin layer, without the need to rub in
- *Proprietary examples include:* Dermamist (white soft paraffin 10%, liquid paraffin, coconut oil); Emollin (liquid paraffin 50%, white soft paraffin 50%)

Additional active ingredients

- Glycerol is a humectant that attracts and retains moisture to hydrate the outer layer of the skin (stratum corneum)
- Urea and lactic acid have keratolytic as well as humectant properties and are useful for very dry and scaling conditions
- Ceramides are physiologic lipids and may improve the emollient effect
- Antiseptic agents (e.g. benzalkonium chloride, chlorhexidine hydrochloride and triclosan) may be useful when there is recurrent skin infection, but are associated with a risk of irritation

or contact allergy. They are therefore most appropriate for use as a soap substitute to be washed off

- Menthol (1–5%) may be effective as symptomatic relief for pruritus

Bath and shower emollients

- Soap and detergent avoidance is a very important part of the management of dry skin and eczema. Bath and shower emollients are widely used to provide a protective lipid layer to the skin surface during bathing. Clinical experience supports their efficacy, though there is no definitive evidence for this

Cautions

- Petrolatum-based emollients are a fire hazard, particularly when used on large body areas. Patients should be warned of this risk

- Use of emollients in the bath or shower makes surfaces more slippery; care should be taken to avoid falls

- Emollients stored in tubs should be removed with a clean spoon or spatula to reduce the risk of bacterial contamination

Common problems

- The emollient effect is short-lived, and repeated applications are essential for maximum benefit. Emollients are often under-prescribed and under-used

- The occlusive nature of ointment-based emollients may cause folliculitis. Emollients should be applied in the direction of hair growth to reduce the risk of folliculitis

- Sodium lauryl sulfate is included as a surfactant or emulsifier in some emollients but may cause

Treatment pearls

- Emollients can be used to 'fill in' fissures, which can reduce pain and speed up healing

- More than one emollient may be required depending on the patient's lifestyle, the severity of the disease, or the time of the day the product is used. For example, a lighter cream preparation may be used during the day and a greasier ointment preparation at night

- Almost any emollient can be used as a soap substitute but there are multiple proprietary preparations, including bath oils and shower gels, which have been designed to make application more convenient

- It is useful to provide a range of products initially in small trial amounts to allow the patient to test acceptability, with the aim of increasing compliance

skin irritation; other additives and preservatives in emollients can induce allergic contact dermatitis

Further reading

Eichenfield LF, Tom WL, Berger TG, et al. Guidelines of care for the management of atopic dermatitis: section 2. Management and treatment of atopic dermatitis with topical therapies. J Am Acad Dermatol 2014; 71:116–132.

Moncrieff G, Cork M, Lawton S, et al. Use of emollients in dry-skin conditions: consensus statement. Clin Exp Dermatol 2013; 38:231–238.

National Institute for Health and Care Excellence. NICE quality standard QS44. Atopic eczema in under 12s. London: NICE, 2013.

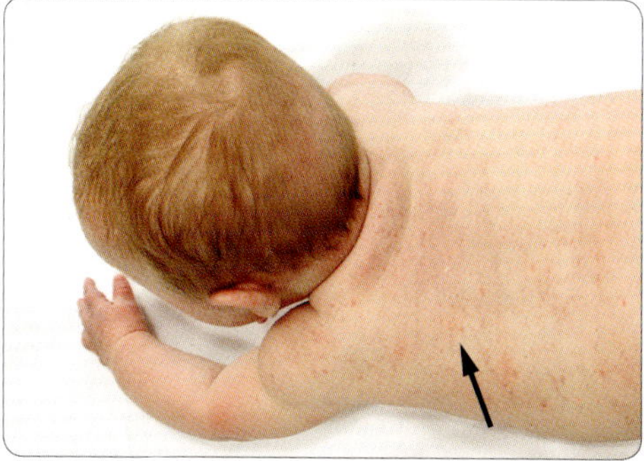

Figure 13.2 Folliculitis is a common complication of greasy emollients, particularly in warm environmental conditions. Treatment includes changing to a water-based preparation. Courtesy of Department of Medical Photography, Ninewells Hospital and Medical School, Dundee.

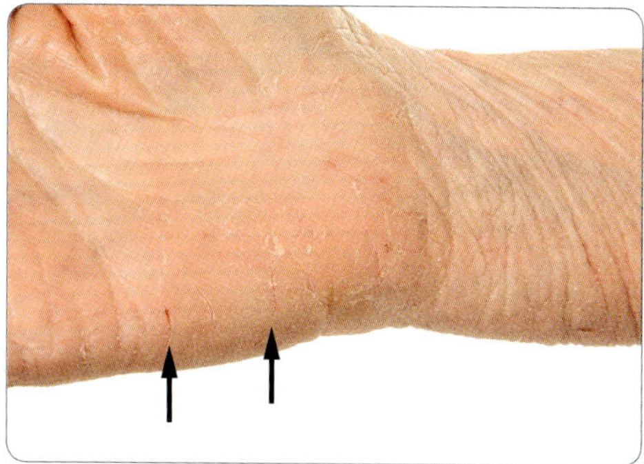

Figure 13.3 Skin fissures can be very painful. Filling the fissure with ointment relieves the pain while softening the epidermal edges to aid healing. Courtesy of Department of Medical Photography, Ninewells Hospital and Medical School, Dundee.

Imiquimod

Dermatologic indications

- Actinic keratoses (face and scalp)
- Superficial basal cell carcinomas < 2 cm
- External genital warts
- *Other reported off-label uses:* Small nodular basal cell carcinomas < 1.5 cm, squamous cell carcinoma in situ (Bowen's disease), lentigo maligna, Porokeratosis of Mibelli, granuloma annulare, extramammary Paget's disease, vulvar intraepithelial neoplasia (VIN), cutaneous T-cell lymphoma, cutaneous melanoma metastases, erythroplasia of Queyrat, morphea, keloids, molluscum contagiosum, pyogenic granuloma

Background

Imiquimod is a synthetic imidazoquinoline amine, which acts as a toll-like receptor-7 (TLR-7) agonist.

It induces activation of nuclear factor-kappa B (NF-κB) and increases transcription and release of interferon-gamma (IFN-γ), tumor necrosis factor-alpha (TNF-α), interferon-alpha (IFN- α), interleukin (IL)-1, -6, -8, -10 and -12, in addition to granulocyte-macrophage colony-stimulating factor and granulocyte colony-stimulating factor.

Imiquimod enhances locally acquired and innate immunity resulting in anti-viral and anti-tumor activity.

Dermatologic prescribing

- Imiquimod cream is available as a 5%, 3.75% or 2.5% preparation
- Imiquimod 5% cream is available as a:
- Box of 12 × 250 mg single-use sachets: one sachet covers an area of 20 cm^2
- 2 g pump pack: four actuations of the pump are equivalent to one 250 mg sachet. The pump lasts 4 weeks once opened (available in Europe, Australia, New Zealand, Canada and Asia)
- Application is a thin layer sparingly to the affected area at night, then washed off with a cleanser and water the following morning
- For actinic keratoses (AKs):
- Imiquimod 5% cream: twice-weekly for 16 weeks (USA)
- Imiquimod 5% cream: thrice-weekly for 4 weeks over 1–2 cycles (4 weeks treatment then 4 weeks rest) (Europe)
- Imiquimod 3.75% or 2.5% cream: once-daily application for 2 weeks, then 2 weeks treatment free, followed by once-daily application for an additional 2 weeks
- For superficial basal cell carcinomas (sBCC):
- Imiquimod 5% cream: once daily five times per week for 6 weeks
- For sBCC, imiquimod should be applied to the the affected area and extended to approximately 1 cm of healthy skin around the edge
- For viral infections including genital warts:
- Imiquimod 5% cream: thrice-weekly for 16 weeks
- About 20 minutes after application, emollients may be applied if necessary

Common problems

- Patients should be educated and given written information regarding the expected local inflammatory reaction as well as potential adverse effects
- Local inflammatory reactions can be severe; they are usually confined to the treatment site, but can extend beyond by a few centimeters
- Expected reactions: erythema, pruritus, burning, and irritation

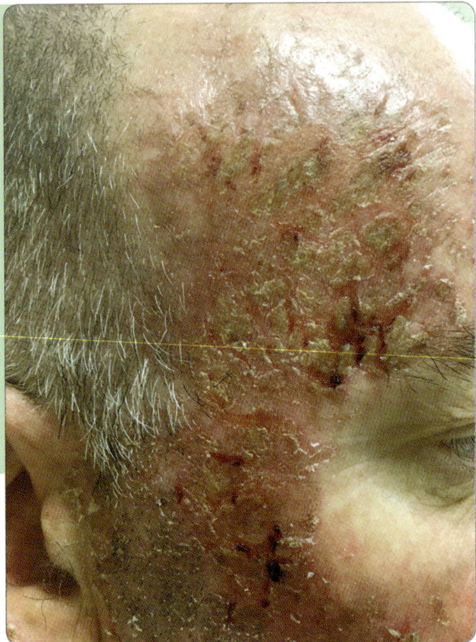

Figure 14.1 Moderately brisk inflammatory reaction (with erythema and crusting) 3 weeks post-commencement of imiquimod for diffuse actinic keratoses/field change.

Treatment pearls

- Instead of storing half-used sachets overnight in the fridge, a pump device may prove more cost-effective for small lesions
- Therapeutic success for superficial BCCs is 80–85%, thus follow-up 3 months after treatment is recommended to confirm cure
- Skin cancers treated non-surgically, e.g. with imiquimod, warrant a minimum of 2 years clinical follow up
- The addition of liquid nitrogen cryotherapy or topical tazarotene or 5-fluorouracil creams may enhance therapeutic success when treating skin cancers
- To treat an entire face or scalp, one to two sachets per application are usually required and at least two boxes per treatment course
- Imiquimod 2–3.75% creams are better tolerated than the 5% cream
- *Immunostimulation:* pre-existing inflammatory arthritis or psoriasis may flare or be unmasked. Episodes of aphthosis, vitiligo, localized psoriasis, pemphigus foliaceus, or vulvar pemphigus may be precipitated
- Although unlicensed, several studies have demonstrated the safe use of imiquimod for the treatment of actinic keratoses and superficial basal cell carcinomas in immunocompromised patients
- *Systemic reactions are uncommon (approximately 1% of patients):* these are flu-like and present with fever, headache, myalgia, fatigue, and regional lymphadenopathy
- Imiquimod should be avoided in pregnancy and breast-feeding.
- *Pigmentary disturbance:* post-inflammatory hypopigmentation or hyperpigmentation are relatively common following treatment
- Off license treatment of molluscum contagiosum: topical imiquimod 5% cream applied thrice-weekly for up to 16 weeks

---

- Less common reactions: vesiculation, erosions, crusting, and ulceration
- Hypopigmented scars can arise in the site of inflammation (which therefore may be larger than the index treated lesion). This complication should be discussed prior to treatment, especially for cosmetically sensitive sites
- Patients should be reassured that the development of an inflammatory reaction predicts therapeutic efficacy
- Treatment may need to temporarily be ceased for a week until the reaction has settled
- If infection is suspected, this should be confirmed microbiologically and treated with appropriate antibiotics
- Severe inflammatory reactions are rare, but more commonly seen in severely sun-damaged skin. Treatment involves ceasing the imiquimod cream, debriding crusts with saline soaks, and considering topical corticosteroids or oral antibiotics

Further reading

Huen AO, Rook AH. Toll receptor agonist therapy of skin cancer and cutaneous T-cell lymphoma. Curr Opin Oncol 2014; 26:237–244.

Micali G, Lacarrubba F, Nasca MR, Schwartz RA. Topical pharmacotherapy for skin cancer: part I. Pharmacology. J Am Acad Dermatol 2014; 70:965.

Micali G, Lacarrubba F, Nasca MR, et al. Topical pharmacotherapy for skin cancer (part II). Clinical applications. J Am Acad Dermatol 2014; 70:979.

Keratolytics

Dermatologic indications

- Keratosis pilaris, ichthyoses, hyperkeratotic skin disorders, eczema, verrucae (viral warts), psoriasis, seborrheic dermatitis, and onychomycosis

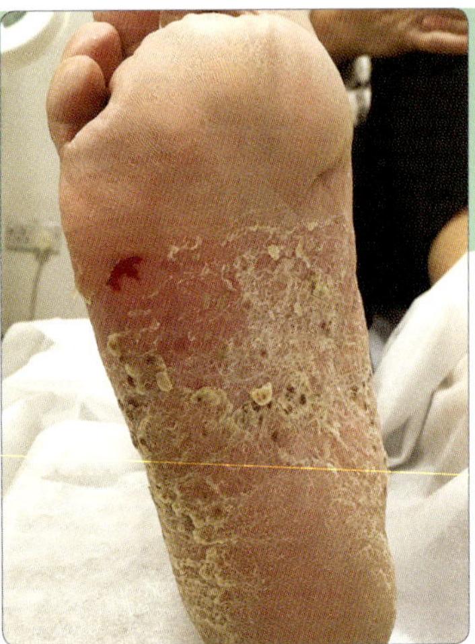

Figure 15.1 Hyperkeratotic pustular dermatosis of the foot.

Background

Topical salicylic acid dissolves thickened skin and scale. It has a wide range of uses in hyperkeratotic skin conditions including keratosis pilaris, ichthyoses, viral warts, psoriasis, and seborrheic dermatitis, amongst others.

Urea cream is a keratin softening and hydrating agent. There are a number of urea containing emollients; these are particularly useful in patients with keratosis pilaris and ichthyoses. It is also frequently used in those with thickened acral skin or palmoplantar keratoderma.

Propylene glycol is an emollient that is often used to aid the penetration of topical corticosteroids. It can be used alone or in combination with urea in the treatment of ichthyoses.

Dermatologic prescribing

Salicylic acid preparations

- Topical salicylic acid preparations designed to treat viral warts are available over the counter in a wide range of concentrations

- Topical salicylic acid dissolved in emulsifying ointment is available in a variety of strengths from 5–50% although these may need to be prepared as special products. They may be useful in severe hyperkeratotic skin disorders, particularly those of the feet

- Betamethasone 0.05% with salicylic acid 3% is used for hyperkeratotic inflammatory dermatoses. It is available as an ointment and a scalp application and used topically once daily to affected areas

- Fluorouracil 0.5% with salicylic acid 10% can be used for hyperkeratotic actinic keratoses. It is applied once daily for up to 12 weeks (see **Chapter 2**). Off-license use for plantar warts has also been reported

- Coal tar solution 12%, salicylic acid 2%, and precipitated sulfur 4% in a coconut oil emollient base is commonly used as a treatment for thick psoriatic plaques on the scalp. It is applied directly to the scalp; initially daily, then weekly

and washed out after 1 hour although some patients can tolerate overnight application

Urea

- Urea containing emollients are applied topically twice daily. A wide range of strengths of urea are available including in combination with lactic acid or ceramides

Propylene glycol, urea and salicylic acid

- Many preparations of propylene glycol, urea, and salicylic acid are not commercially available. These require compounding at specialist pharmacies, which can be expensive. In addition, concerns regarding the standard and quality of products have been raised. Multiple compounded keratolytic products are summarized in **Table 15.1**

Cautions

- Salicylic acid should not be used on the face or genital skin or in individuals with peripheral neuropathy or impaired circulation

- Salicylic acid used in neonates or applied to large body surface areas may result in salicylic acid toxicity and should be avoided

- Avoid concomitant oral and topical salicylates use in neonates or on large body surface areas due to risk of salicylate toxicity

- Contact allergy to propylene glycol may develop

Table 15.1 Unlicensed dermatologic preparations that can be compounded in specialist pharmacies

Preparation	Clinical use
Salicylic acid (2–20%) in emulsifying ointment	Soften hyperkeratosis in any hyperkeratotic skin disorder
Propylene glycol 20% in aqueous cream	Emollient in very dry skin disorders
Propylene glycol 40% in clobetasol propionate 0.05% cream	Severe inflammatory dermatoses without hyperkeratosis or sensitive skin sites
Salicylic acid 5%, propylene glycol 47.5% in clobetasol propionate 0.05%	Severe hyperkeratotic eczema, palmoplantar pustulosis, and psoriasis
Coal tar solution BP 3.3%, propylene glycol 20% in fluocinolone acetonide 0.025%	Inflammatory hyerkeratotic scalp psoriasis
Zinc and salicylic acid paste (Lassar's paste) half-strength	Irritant and/or flexural dermatitis, hand dermatitis, and exudative eczematous conditions
Salicylic acid 2% and sulfur 2% in aqueous cream	Scaly inflammatory skin disorders of the face
Coconut oil 25% in emulsifying ointment	Severe scaling of the scalp

Adapted from Specials Recommended by the British Association of Dermatologists for Skin Disease, 2014

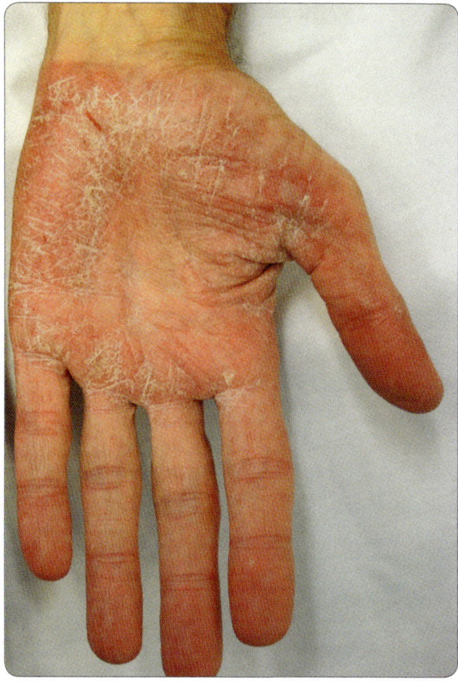

Figure 15.2 Hyperkeratotic hand eczema. Note fissuring on the hypothenar eminence.

Common problems

- Viral warts must be regularly pared down using a pumice stone or file between salicylic acid applications for treatment to be effective. Care must be taken not to get salicylic acid on the surrounding normal skin as this can cause skin irritation; white soft paraffin can be used to protect the surrounding skin

- Patients must continue treatment for at least 3 months; lack of patient compliance is a common reason for treatment failure

- Topical treatments for scalp psoriasis can be very challenging for an individual to apply alone. The hair must be carefully and systematically parted for the treatment to be applied to the scalp in order for it to be effective

> **Treatment pearls**
>
> - Use a tar-based shampoo to wash out salicylic acid scalp preparations
> - Keratolytics should not be applied to fissured or ulcerated skin as they will cause pain

Further reading

Buckley D, Root T, Bath S. Specials Recommended by the British Association of Dermatologists for Skin Disease. London: British Association of Dermatologists, 2014.

Kwok CS, Gibbs S, Bennett C, Holland R, Abbott R. Topical treatments for cutaneous warts. Cochrane Database Syst Rev 2012;9:CD001781.

Minoxidil

Dermatologic indications

- Male and female pattern hair loss (androgenetic alopecia)

Background

2% minoxidil solution and 5% minoxidil foam are approved for female pattern hair loss.

5% minoxidil, as solution or foam, is approved for the treatment of male pattern hair loss.

Minoxidil is a potassium channel opener and vasodilator. Its mode of action in androgenetic alopecia remains unclear.

In animal studies, topical minoxidil induces telogen hairs to enter the anagen phase and may also prolong anagen duration, thus increasing follicle size and reversing miniaturization.

In humans, topical minoxidil increases hair count and weight.

Dermatologic prescribing

- Minoxidil should be applied as 1 mL of solution or half a cap of foam to affected areas on the scalp once (5% minoxidil for women) or twice (2% minoxidil for women and 5% for men) daily

- The hair and scalp must be dry before application, and minoxidil should be left in place for at least 4 hours

- Treatment efficacy should be assessed at least 6 months after starting treatment

- Treatment should be continued to maintain the efficacy

- A review of treatments for female pattern hair loss concluded that a greater proportion of participants treated with minoxidil reported a moderate increase in their hair regrowth compared with placebo (relative risk 1.86, 95% confidence interval 1.42-2.43)

- The original trials of minoxidil in men showed large placebo effects. Much of the regrowth observed following minoxidil use is fine, cosmetically insignificant hairs. Experts have suggested the following real outcomes following minoxidil use: 15% experience medium regrowth, 50% have their hair loss delayed, and 35% continue to lose hair

Cautions

- Systemic absorption of minoxidil through the skin is minimal, but palpitations and hypotension have been reported

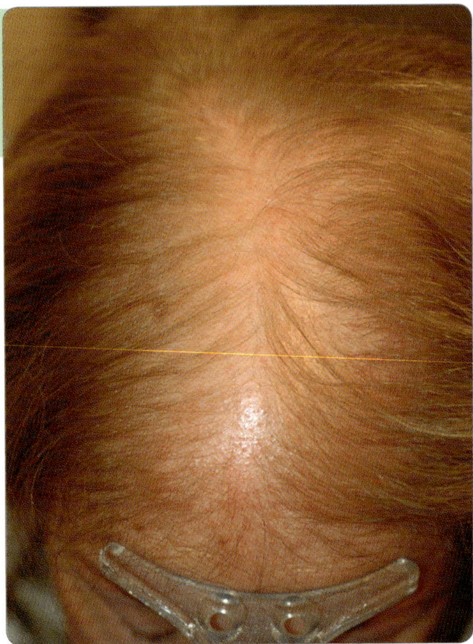

Figure 16.1 Woman with frontal accentuation of female pattern hair loss (courtesy of Dr Jerry Shapiro).

Common problems

- Hypertrichosis of the forehead and face is a possible side effect and is more common with the 5% concentration

- A temporary increase in hair shedding may occur upon initiation of minoxidil treatment. Patients should be counseled regarding this potential side effect and treatment should be discontinued if increased hair shedding persists for > 2 weeks

- Headaches

Further reading

Blumeyer A, Tosti A, Messenger A, et al. Evidence-based (S3) guideline for the treatment of androgenetic alopecia in women and in men. J Dtsch Dermatol Ges 2011; 9:S1–57.

Georgala S, Befon A, Maniatopoulou E, Georgala C. Topical use of minoxidil in children and systemic side effects. Dermatology 2007; 214:101–102.

Messenger AG, Rundegren J. Minoxidil: mechanisms of action on hair growth. Br J Dermatol 2004; 150:186–194.

Sinclair R. Male pattern androgenetic alopecia. Br Med J 1998; 317:865–869.

van Zuuren EJ1, Fedorowicz Z, Carter B. Evidence-based treatments for female pattern hair loss: a summary of a Cochrane systematic review. Br J Dermatol 2012; 167:995–1010.

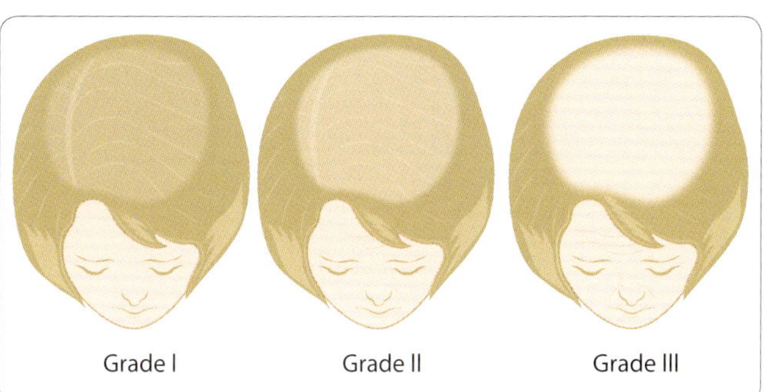

Figure 16.2 Ludwig scale for female pattern hair loss.

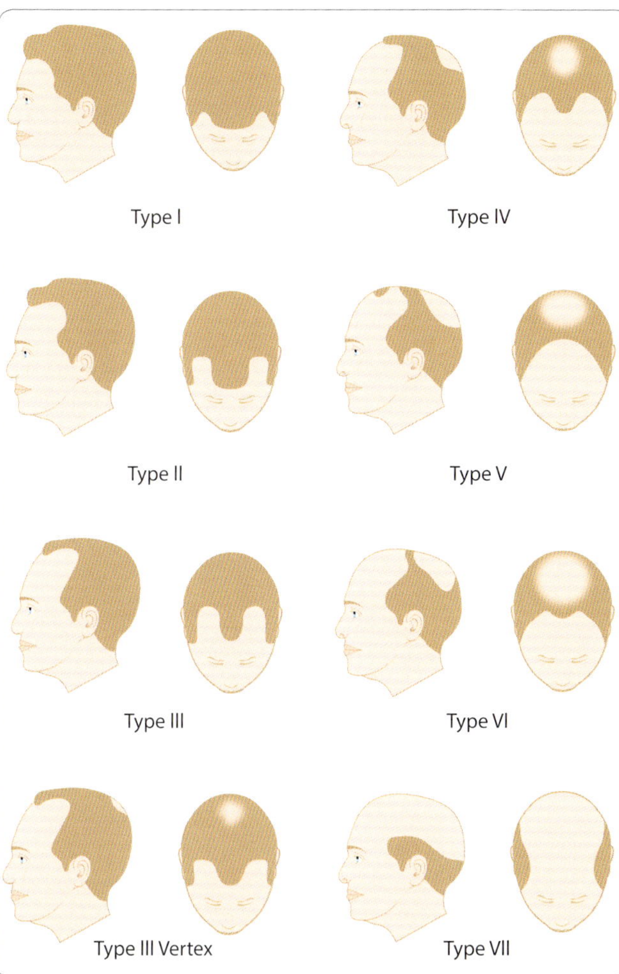

Figure 16.3 Norwood scale for male pattern hair loss.

Treatment pearls

- Irritant and allergic contact dermatitis may occur and are usually related to the solution vehicle, propylene glycol, which can be avoided by use of the 5% foam

- Patients should be encouraged to apply minoxidil at least 2 hours before going to bed to avoid contamination of the pillow, with subsequent facial contact and potential unwanted hair growth

- Patients should be counseled that cessation of minoxidil will result in loss of the hair gained from its use; hence, application should be continued for life or until the patient no longer desires the beneficial effects of minoxidil

Retinoids

Dermatologic indications

- Acne, psoriasis, hyperpigmentation, melasma, solar lentigines, photo-aging, fine wrinkles (rhytids)
- Less commonly used for actinic keratoses, keratosis pilaris, hypertrophic scars, and Darier's disease
- May have a role in wound healing
- *Topical alitretinoin:* Kaposi's sarcoma, palmar hyperkeratosis
- *Topical bexarotene:* cutaneous T-cell lymphoma

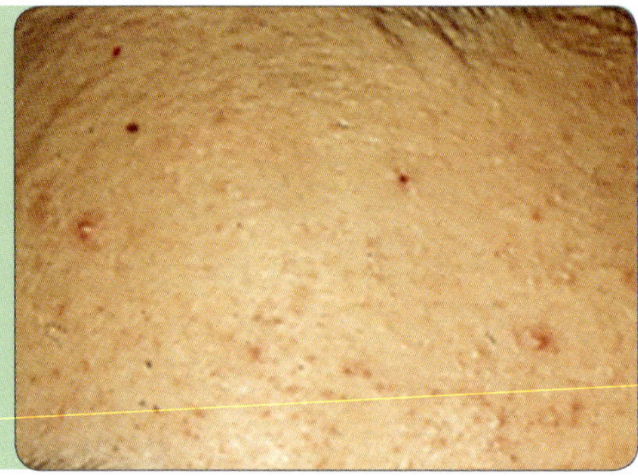

Figure 17.1 Comedonal and pustular acne (grade 1) responds best to a topical retinoid/ antibiotic combination or a topical retinoid/ benzoyl peroxide combination. Both combinations can be irritants to the skin causing erythema, scaling, and dryness. Tolerance to topical retinoids can be built up with twice weekly application initially, increasing to daily application after several weeks.

Background

Retinoids are vitamin A derivatives.

Tretinoin (all-trans-retinoic acid) is a first generation synthetic retinoid.

Isotretinoin (13-cis retinoic acid) is an isomer of tretinoin that is more photostable and associated with less skin irritation.

Adapalene and tazarotene represent synthetic, third-generation retinoids.

The retinoid class of topical agents act on keratinocytes and normalize hyperkeratinization.

In acne, retinoids prevent the formation of microcomedos, the precursor lesion in inflammatory acne. The use of topical retinoids in acne also promotes an indirect antimicrobial effect through promoting a more aerobic environment (see **Chapter 1**).

Tretinoin/retinoic acid and isotretinoin aid in the treatment of photoaging through limitation of UV-induced degradation of the dermal matrix and an increase in the production of procollagen.

Dermatologic prescribing

- Patient support and education are essential during retinoid therapy to ensure successful clinical outcomes
- Acne:
- Topical retinoids for acne are available in cream, gel, and liquid forms. Creams can be less irritating than gel or liquid forms
- Adapalene 0.1% gel is biologically equivalent to tretinoin 0.025% gel
- Topical retinoids work best on comedonal acne using once daily (at night) application of tretinoin, adapalene, adapalene combined with benzoyl peroxide, or isotretinoin
- The combination of a retinoid with a topical antibiotic (erythromycin or clindamycin applied nightly) is useful for mild papular/pustular acne

- Moderate inflammatory acne can be treated with an oral antibiotic and topical retinoid or retinoid/benzoyl peroxide combination
- Psoriasis:
- Tazarotene gel applied nightly for up to 3 months, to treat small areas of chronic, mild-to-moderate plaque psoriasis
- To limit problems with irritation, short term regimens with topical corticosteroids used once daily or on alternate days in combination with tazarotene may be effective
- Melasma:
- Combination therapy with hydroquinone, tretinoin, and hydrocortisone (Pigmanorm) or fluocinolone acetonide 0.01% (Triluma) applied nightly for 3–6 months
- It is essential to combine this treatment regimen with year-round broad spectrum, high factor UV protection
- Actinic keratoses:
- Adapalene applied nightly to superficial actinic keratoses and field change for at least 6 months reduces the degree of actinic damage and the number of actinic keratoses

Cautions

- Retinoids are highly teratogenic
- Although absorption of topical retinoids leads to much lower systemic concentrations than oral preparations, routine use of topical

retinoids is contraindicated during pregnancy or lactation

■ If pregnancy occurs during topical retinoid use, the topical therapy should be discontinued immediately. Women of child-bearing age should be counseled regarding the risks of retinoid use during pregnancy

Common problems

■ 'Retinoid dermatitis' is common, resulting in:

● Burning or itching

● Excessive dryness and scaling of the skin

● Erythema

■ In order to alleviate retinoid dermatitis, changes in application form (creams less irritating than gels/liquids), concentration, amount, or frequency are usually effective

■ By thinning the stratum corneum, retinoids reduce natural photoprotection, which can lead to photosensitivity

■ Less common problems include:

● Swelling or peeling of the skin

● Initial flare of acne as the comedones and deeper microcomedones are extruded through the epidermis

● An initial flare of eczema can occur in those with a history of eczema

● Blistering

Further reading

Jones DA. The potential immunomodulatory effects of topical retinoids. Dermatol Online J 2005; 11:3.

Thielitz A, Gollnick H. Topical retinoids in acne vulgaris: update on efficacy and safety. Am J Clin Dermatol 2008; 9:369–381.

Vahlquist A, Duvic M (Eds). Retinoids and carotenoids in dermatology. Boca Raton, FL: CRC Press, 2007.

Treatment pearls

■ Acne usually requires several months of treatment to show significant improvement

■ It should be explained to the patient that they will experience drying of the skin

■ Topical retinoids should be applied to completely dry skin to minimize irritation

■ Topical retinoids should be applied at night as they are deactivated by sunlight

■ Topical retinoids should be applied on alternate nights or even as little as twice weekly at first, slowly escalating to nightly applications as tolerated

■ Sunscreen applied in the morning reduces problems with photosensitivity

■ Cosmetics and gentle cleansers or non-oil based moisturisers may be used; there is no need to amend the frequency of washing or application of moisturizer because of the topical retinoid treatment. Harsh astringents should be avoided to minimize irritation

■ Tazarotene should not be used for flexural psoriasis as it is likely to cause substantial irritation

Dermatologic indications

- *Permethrin 5% cream:* scabies and pediculosis pubis
- *Malathion 0.5% lotion:* scabies, pediculosis capitis, pediculosis pubis
- *Benzyl benzoate 25% lotion:* scabies
- *Oral ivermectin:* strongyloidiasis and onchocerciasis (US), strongyloidiasis and scabies (France), no licensed indications (UK)
- *Oral ivermectin:* scabies and cutaneous larva migrans
- *Topical ivermectin 1% cream:* licensed for the treatment of rosacea

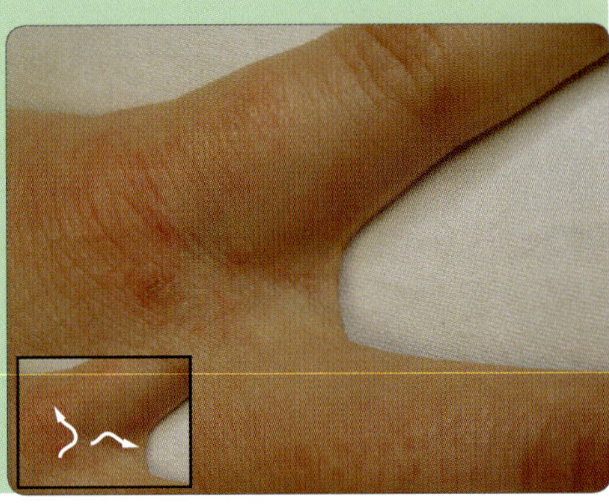

Figure 18.1 Finger web showing two scabies burrows. Inset shows the track of the burrow (arrowheads at burrow end where the mite can be located).

Background

Scabies is a contagious, intensely pruritic dermatosis caused by the mite *Sarcoptes scabiei var. hominis*. The incubation period is usually 2–6 weeks but may be as long as 2 months or may be much shorter in cases of re-infestation.

Symptoms of scabies are caused by a hypersensitivity to the mite, and pruritus is often reported to be worse at night.

Transmission is from person-to-person through close skin-to-skin contact although occasionally fomites are implicated.

Scabies is common in children, particularly in resource limited settings, but is also seen in institutional settings such as boarding schools, residential care facilities, and prisons. It is also more prevalent in pregnant women and breastfeeding mothers.

The mite may be visualised directly using a dermatoscope or with a microscope following removal from a burrow with a needle.

Chronic, heavy infestation may lead to a hyperkeratotic form known as crusted scabies in which pruritus may be mild or absent. Crusted scabies may be associated with the immunosuppression of HIV or HTLV-1 infection.

Dermatologic prescribing

- It is essential to treat both symptomatic individuals and their close contacts simultaneously to prevent re-infestation
- Topical agents should be applied to the entire skin surface although in adults, treatment of the face and scalp is usually unnecessary
- *Malathion 0.5% lotion:* two applications administered 7 days apart. Leave on for 24 hours
- *Permethrin 5% cream:* one application left on for 8–12 hours. Treatment should be repeated after 7 days
- *Benzyl benzoate 25% lotion:* one treatment applied on 3 days consecutively. It is advisable to dilute in children to 12.5% or 6.25%
- *Ivermectin 200 µg/kg body weight:* taken orally as a single dose, which may be repeated. Resistance has been reported
- Managing scabies in very young infants is challenging and specialist advice should

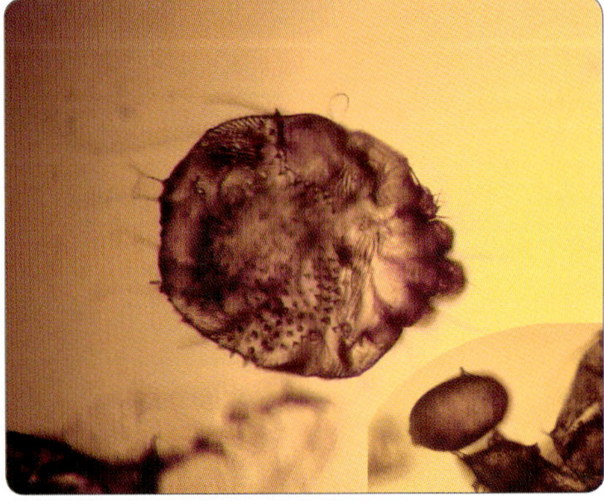

Figure 18.2 Microscopy showing scabies mite, and scabies egg (inset) x 50.

Treatment pearls

- Treatment failure is most likely to be due to adherence issues rather than primary resistance of the mite

- Mites may be present under the nails. The nails should be trimmed and topical treatment should be applied to this area

- Patients should be advised to reapply topical therapy after hand washing

- There is no consensus on the treatment of crusted scabies, however, many would advocate the use of oral ivermectin in conjunction with repeated applications of a topical scabicide

- Keratolytics such as 2% salicylic acid ointment may be a useful adjunct in crusted scabies

- There is no consensus on how to manage fomites including bedding. Normal laundry practices for bed linen, towels, and clothing should take place at the time of treatment. Some authors advocate washing items at a temperature of $\geq 50°C$, especially for items associated with individuals diagnosed with crusted scabies. Items that are difficult to wash can be placed in a sealed plastics bags for 3 days

- Urinalysis should be performed in children with scabies with secondary bacterial sepsis because of the association with post-streptococcal glomerulonephritis

- Sexual health screening should be considered in those who may have acquired the condition from a sexual partner

- Other topical agents for scabies include Lindane 1% lotion, sulfur 10% ointment, and crotamiton 10% cream or lotion. Their use is limited by one or more of the following: availability, toxicity, low effectiveness

- Ivermectin 1% cream has been reported to be effective in the treatment of scabies

be sought. Permethrin 5% cream is not recommended under 2 months of age. Malathion 0.5% is not recommended until the age of 6 months. The safety of oral ivermectin in children weighing less than 15 kg has not been established

- Permethrin 5% cream and malathion 0.5% lotion appear to be safe to use during pregnancy and in women who are breastfeeding

Common problems

- Healthcare workers often prescribe insufficient quantities of topical agents

- Ensuring that household or other significant contacts receive treatment is often difficult

- Pruritus may persist for weeks following successful eradication of the mite and may require treatment with oral anti-histamines, emollients, crotamiton 10% cream, or topical corticosteroids. It is important, but sometimes difficult, to distinguish this persistent itch from scabies treatment failure

- Benzyl benzoate is more of an irritant than malathion or permethrin

- Benzyl benzoate 25% lotion is not available in the US. It is available in the UK but not recommended. However, it is on the World Health Organization's List of Essential Medicines

- Permethrin is available as a 1% lotion to treat head lice, but is ineffective in the treatment of scabies in this form. This leads to errors in prescribing

Further reading

Scott GR, Chosidow O. European Guideline for the Management of Scabies, 2010. Int J STD AIDS 2011; 22:301-303.

Chosidow O. Clinical practices. Scabies. N Engl J Med 2006; 354:1718–1727.

Golant AK, Levitt JO. Scabies: a review of diagnosis and management based on mite biology. Pediatr Rev 2012; 33:e1-e12.

Dermatologic indications

- Alopecia areata
- Resistant viral warts

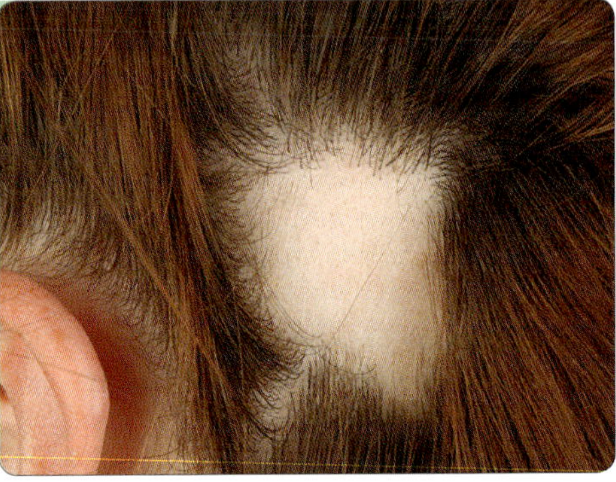

Figure 19.1 Patchy alopecia areata.

Background

Diphencyprone (DPCP) is a potent contact sensitizer and the most common contact immunotherapeutic agent.

Ultraviolet (UV) light causes degradation of the chemical. DPCP is therefore prepared in acetone, which prevents this process.

The mechanism of induction of allergic contact dermatitis to DPCP follows the classical pathway of sensitization. It is likely that DPCP is haptenated by host proteins to form a chemical antigen which is presented by cutaneous dendritic cells to T-cells in the draining lymph node. Antigen-specific T-cells (mostly CD8+) undergo population expansion and recirculate to the skin. On re-exposure to DPCP, at the skin surface, cutaneous dendritic cells (and possibly keratinocytes) present DPCP to DPCP-specific T-cells causing cytokine release and inflammation. It is thought that this immune stimulation may 'distract' the anti-follicular CD8+ response which is responsible for inducing alopecia areata.

Dermatologic prescribing

- DPCP is often used in patients with alopecia totalis (loss of all scalp hair) in whom injected steroid treatment is not possible due to the large area involved.

- The patient is initially sensitized with 2% DPCP solution on a small area of the scalp. The treatment is subsequently commenced by applying 0.001% DPCP solution, followed by weekly application of increasing concentrations of DPCP until a mild eczematous reaction/contact dermatitis is obtained. Concentrations commonly used are 0.001%, 0.005%, 0.01%, 0.1%, 0.5%, 1% and 1.5%

- Once the concentration of DPCP that produces a moderate eczematous reaction has been established, the treatment can be applied to the affected areas every week or fortnight until complete hair regrowth is achieved. Treatment intervals will then slowly decrease and eventually stop

- The treated area should not be washed or exposed to sunlight for 48 hours

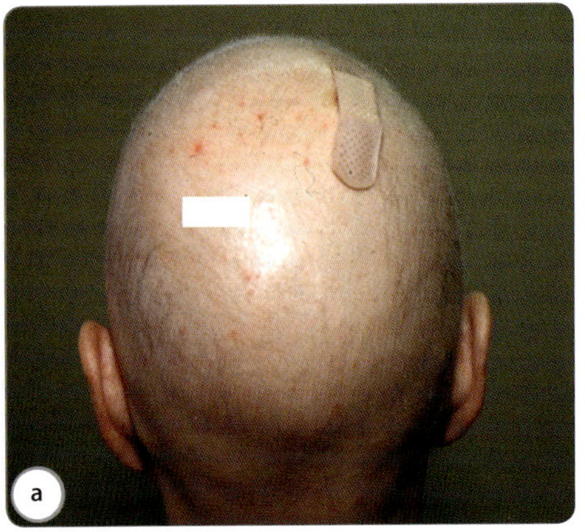

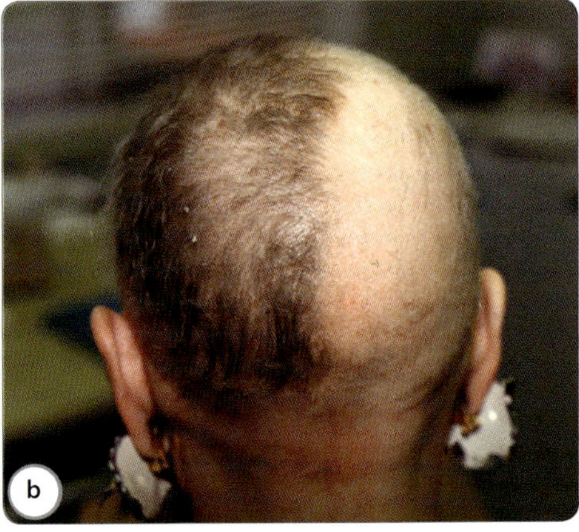

Figure 19.2 A female patient with alopecia totalis before (a) and after (b) treatment with DPCP (courtesy of Dr Jerry Shapiro).

- The minimum treatment duration is between 3–6 months. If there is no response within this timeframe, the patient is considered to be a non-responder
- 1–2% of patients develop a tolerance against DPCP and fail to sensitize even after 2% DPCP application
- A clinically significant response is produced in 30% of patients after 6 months. Some evidence suggests that the response rate is improved with more prolonged treatment

Cautions

- This treatment is not recommended in pregnancy or lactation
- Patients should avoid sunbathing or using tanning beds while having DPCP treatment

Common problems

- Generalized eczema (1–40% of patients) or urticarial reactions (2–10%)
- Vitiligo occurs in 7% of patients treated with DPCP
- Local blistering and swelling
- Regional lymphadenopathy may occur
- Both hypo- and hyperpigmentation may develop at the treatment site

Treatment pearls

- The contact allergen can be washed off early if the patient experiences an overwhelming contact dermatitis. The patient should have a potent topical corticosteroid available for use during the treatment period
- The patient should wear a hat following treatment to protect the area from exposure to sunlight
- Treatment is often initially applied to one half of the scalp and only applied to both sides after the treated side has shown substantial hair re-growth

Further reading

Blume-Peytavi U, Tosti A, Whitting DA, Trüeb RM (Eds). Hair growth and disorders. Berlin: Springer-Verlag, 2008.

Buckley DA, Du Vivier AW. The therapeutic use of topical contact sensitizers in benign dermatoses. Br J Dermatol 2001; 145:385–405.

Hoffmann R, Happle R. Topical immunotherapy in alopecia areata. What, how, and why? Dermatol Clin 1996; 14:739–744.

Rokhsar CK, Shupack JL, Vafai JJ et al. Efficacy of topical sensitizers in the treatment of alopecia areata. J Am Acad Dermatol 1998; 39:751 -61.

Sunscreens

Dermatologic indications

- Photo-sensitive skin disorders such as polymorphic light eruption or solar urticaria
- Photo-exacerbated disorders such as discoid lupus erythematosus, dermatomyositis, rosacea, chronic actinic dermatitis
- Skin cancer prevention, especially in patients on immunosuppressive drugs such as azathioprine or cyclosporine
- Prevention and treatment of actinic keratoses/field change
- Personal use: to prevent sunburn, for activities in the sun, and to reduce the risk of photoaging

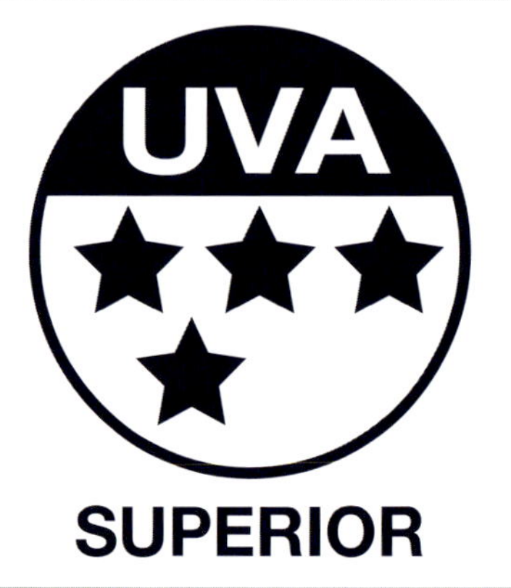

Figure 20.1 Sunscreen labelling indicating good UVA protection.

Background

Sunscreens are designed to reduce skin exposure to ultraviolet B (UVB), ultraviolet A (UVA), and sometimes visible light. UVA protection is more critical for: photocarcinogenesis, photoaging and drug photosensitizers (usually); UVB protection is more critical for the prevention of sunburn; both are important for photosensitive dermatoses

'Reflectant' sunscreens

- These contain micronized titanium dioxide or zinc oxide; these products appear white to variable degrees on the skin
- Approximately 50% of sunscreen products contain titanium dioxide as well as absorbent chemicals
- Although an effective sunblock, titanium dioxide contributes to the 'whiteness' following application. High concentrations of titanium dioxide are often used in sporting environments

'Absorbent' sunscreens

- These contain chemicals that absorb ultraviolet radiation
- These may be primarily UVA, UVB, or broad-spectrum absorbers. Of the 26 sunscreen chemicals permitted for use in the EU, 19 were found in a 2011 survey of sunscreen products in the UK. Fewer sunscreen chemicals are permitted for use in the US
- Some are widely used: butyl methoxydibenzoylmethane and octocrylene, for example, were found in > 90% of products. On average, a sunscreen will contain approximately five absorbent chemicals

Sun protection factor

- This is a measure of protection provided against burning, compared to unprotected skin. It mainly represents UVB protection
- SPF30 should enable a person to stay 30 times longer in the sun without burning than would be the case if no sunscreen were applied. However, manufacturer-quoted SPF values are measured using a far higher surface density of sunscreen application than is achieved in reality, and only 50% or less of the quoted SPF is typically likely to be achieved in normal use
- There is no industry-standardized method of measuring or declaring protection against UVA. A star rating system is often used, with a 4- or 5-star product offering good UVA protection, sometimes also indicated by the letters 'UVA' surrounded by a circle (**Figure 20.1**)

Dermatologic prescribing

- For medical use (i.e. disease prevention), sunscreens with an SPF of at least 30 and with good UVA protection should be recommended
- The product should be applied liberally before exposure, with a further application soon afterwards to ensure adequate surface density and to treat any areas potentially missed when first applied
- Sunscreen should be reapplied after swimming or sweating
- Tinted reflectant-only sunscreens are available, which provide some protection against visible light as well as ultraviolet light, and are useful for patients with severe photosensitivity including porphyria-induced photosensitivity

- Sunscreens containing absorbent chemicals are not recommended for use in infants, where protection through strict sun avoidance is preferred, or use of a titanium dioxide product if necessary

Common problems

- Skin irritation, particularly when applied to areas prone to eczema
- Reflectant sunscreens are generally less irritating than absorbent sunscreens
- Patients should be encouraged to try various formulations well before their vacation
- Acne, usually of the face, is common in acne-prone individuals. In these cases, reduced use of sunscreens and increased sun avoidance is recommended
- Contact dermatitis to sunscreens, particularly absorbent sunscreens, may occur. This adverse effect is important to recognize as it may be severe and can be misdiagnosed as an idiopathic photodermatosis, such as polymorphic light eruption or chronic actinic dermatitis
- Most of the allergic reactions to sunscreen chemicals are 'photocontact', requiring both application to the skin and then sunlight exposure to induce the problem
- This adverse effect may be investigated by photopatch testing, where sunscreen chemicals are applied as patch tests, then exposed 24 hours later to a small dose of UVA, with the final reading being made 72 or 96 hours after application

Treatment pearls

- Sunscreens are usually less efficient at blocking UVA compared with UVB, therefore extended use may allow an unnaturally high dose of UVA
- This should be avoided in photosensitive eruptions and in prevention of skin malignancy
- Instead, sunscreen combined with wide-brimmed hats and sun-protective clothing as well as reduced sun exposure duration should be recommended
- Sunscreen chemicals are found in a wide range of cosmetic products including lip salves, face creams, and some shampoos. Patients who are allergic to specific sunscreen chemicals should be alerted to this potential risk of exposure
- 'Hypoallergenic' sunscreens do not, in general, differ from other available products
- Sunscreens marketed for children often contain a similar number of absorbent chemicals as other products, but are more likely to contain titanium dioxide

Further reading

Kerr AC. A survey of the availability of sunscreen filters in the UK. Clin Exp Dermatol 2011; 36:541–543.

Linos E, Keiser E, Fu T, et al. Hat, shade, long sleeves, or sunscreen? Rethinking US sun protection messages based on their relative effectiveness. Cancer Causes Control 2011; 22:1067-1071.

Tars

Dermatologic indications

- Psoriasis
- Eczematous dermatoses
- Pruritus

Background

Tars are distillation products of organic material. Tars derived from wood, shale, and especially coal, have been used in the treatment of skin disease for many centuries.

Tars can contain thousands of constituents, which will vary somewhat depending on the exact source, temperature of distillation, and subsequent processing. They are not chemically standardized, and the active constituents are not firmly established.

Coal tar contains polycyclic aromatic hydrocarbons, which are known to be absorbed through the skin to some degree. However the theoretical risks of carcinogenicity have not been evident in practice.

Dermatologic prescribing

- Coal tar solution a constituent of many commercial formulations, contains 20% coal tar
- Coal tar, combined with ultraviolet B (UVB) light is the basis of the traditional Goeckerman regimen for psoriasis, which has also been adapted for atopic dermatitis. Daily treatment with UVB (narrowband for psoriasis) followed by applications of 2–5% crude coal tar have been reported to achieve 100% PASI75 at week 12
- Some dermatologic products contain other tars such as wood and shale tars. Wood tars include beech, birch, and pine oils as well as cade oil (extracted from juniper). Shale tar is also known as ichthammol or ichthyol. These tars are often less irritating than coal tar and are much less likely to photosensitize
- Cade oil is a constituent of many shampoos used for the treatment of scalp dermatoses
- More highly refined tar products such as Exorex lotion are available which have less odor
- Coal tar shampoos are commonly used for scalp psoriasis along with tar and salicylic acid preparations such as Cocois or Sebco

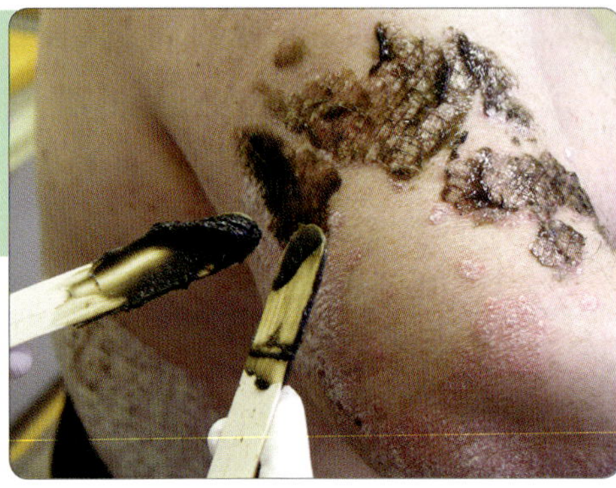

Figure 21.1 Application of 2% crude coal tar in yellow soft paraffin to treat psoriasis (note that the nurse is wearing gloves).

Common problems

- The smell of coal tar is attractive to some, but offensive to many patients
- Crude coal tar is a messy and inconvenient treatment, and is often impractical for patients to apply at home. Tar extracts are generally more acceptable, but may still stain clothing
- Coal tar may be an irritant, especially when used in flexures or on facial skin
- Folliculitis is commonly observed following use
- Coal tar is photosensitizing (to UVA and visible light), and patients must be warned that sun exposure during tar therapy may result in severe unexpected burning. However, when carefully dosed and monitored, tar and UVB can be used very effectively in combination
- On occasion, wood tars can induce allergic sensitization resulting in contact dermatitis. This seems to be rarely observed with coal tar

Further reading

Dennis M, Bhutani T, Koo J, Liao W. Goeckerman therapy for the treatment of eczema: a practical guide and review of efficacy. J Dermatol Treat 2013; 24:2–6.

Goeckerman WH. Treatment of psoriasis. Arch Dermatol Syphilol 1931; 24:446–450.

Goodfield M, Kownacki S, Berth-Jones J. Double-blind, randomised, multicentre, parallel group study comparing a 1% coal tar preparation (Exorex) with a 5% coal tar preparation (Alphosyl) in chronic plaque psoriasis. J Dermatol Treat 2004; 15:14–22.

Lebwohl MG, Heymann WR, Berth-Jones J, Coulson I (Eds). Treatment of skin disease: comprehensive therapeutic strategies, 4th Edn. Philadelphia: Elsevier Saunders, 2014.

Lee E, Koo J. Modern modified 'ultra' Goeckerman therapy: a PASI assessment of a very effective therapy for psoriasis resistant to both prebiologic and biologic therapies. J Dermatol Treat 2005;16:102–107.

Treatment pearls

- Crude coal tar is an effective treatment for psoriasis. Before topical corticosteroids were introduced, tar was a mainstay in the treatment of eczema
- The efficacy of tar-containing products such as shampoos and bath additives is less well established
- Tar needs prolonged skin contact, for several hours daily, in order to work well. Short applications are generally ineffective
- Overnight application, while wearing old clothes including gloves and socks as required, can be a practical approach for some patients. Alternatively, a range of tubular bandages can be used
- Tar is often used with coconut oil for scalp psoriasis, and is best applied overnight, covered with a shower cap, and washed off in the morning
- Tar often works well for small plaque and guttate psoriasis, which can be difficult to treat with dithranol, as it is impossible to avoid contaminating normal skin. Low tar concentrations ($\leq 2\%$) should be used initially
- Ichthammol (shale tar) or coal tar may be applied in paste bandages and can be very soothing, relieving pruritus in atopic dermatitis (atopic eczema) or other eczematous eruptions. Instruction by a trained and skilled nurse is required for best results
- As with all topical therapy, optimal results are obtained from inpatient care, but well-supervised application of tar by experienced nurses in a dermatology outpatient unit is almost as effective. The results of self-treatment at home are highly dependent on the dedication of the patient

Vitamin D analogs

Dermatologic indications

- Psoriasis (plaque, flexural)
- *Also used for:* alopecia areata, morphea, palmoplantar pustulosis, ichthyosis, keratoderma, Grover's disease, disseminated superficial porokeratosis, Hailey–Hailey disease, lichen slcerosus, pityriasis rubra pilaris, acanthosis nigricans (unlicensed)

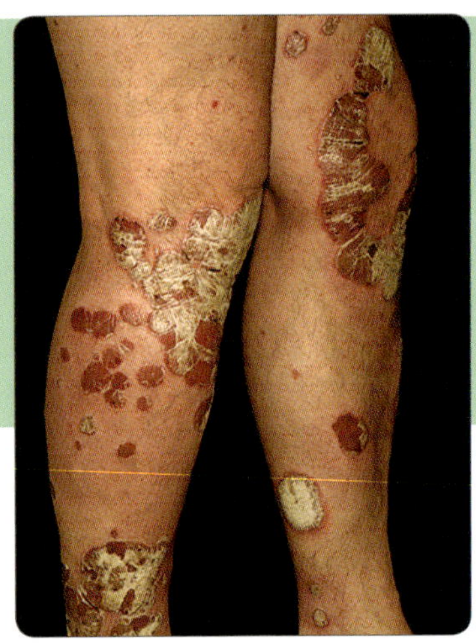

Figure 22.1 Vitamin D analogs are commonly prescribed for the treatment of plaque psoriasis.

Background

Calcitriol, the active metabolite of vitamin D, and two vitamin D analogs, calcipotriol and tacalcitol are frequently used in the treatment of psoriasis and less commonly used for other skin conditions.

These drugs bind to vitamin D receptors which in turn bind to vitamin D response elements on target genes, resulting in inhibition of cellular proliferation and inflammation, immunomodulation, as well as induction of differentiation; all key components known to be dysregulated in psoriasis.

Vitamin D analogs are often used in combination with potent topical corticosteroids as first-line topical therapy for psoriasis.

Dermatologic prescribing

- Vitamin D analogs are relatively easy to apply and are cosmetically acceptable to most patients
- They do not smell or stain the skin, unlike coal tar and dithranol preparations, respectively: this may be particularly important in 'high impact' sites including the face, flexures, and scalp
- Preparations, frequency, and maximum weekly dose varies within this class
- Calcipotriol (available as ointment and solution):
  - Once or twice daily
  - Up to 5000 µg per week (e.g. 70 g of 50 mg/g ointment per week + 30 mL of 50 mg/mL scalp solution)
- Calcitriol (available as ointment):
  - Twice daily
  - Up to 630 mg per week (e.g. 210 g of 3 mg/g ointment)
- Tacalcitol (available as ointment and lotion):
  - Once daily preferably at bedtime
  - Up to 280 mg per week (e.g. 40 g of 4 mg/g ointment + 30 mL of 4 mg/mL lotion)

Cautions

- *Pregnancy and lactation risks:* advice varies within this class
- *Calcipotriol:* should be avoided in pregnancy unless essential; no information in lactation.
- *Calcitriol:* should only be used in restricted amounts in pregnancy if clearly necessary; monitor serum and urine calcium concentration. Should be avoided in lactation
- *Tacalcitol:* no information is available in pregnancy or lactation, but the manufacturer recommends avoiding the breast area when breastfeeding
- *Calcium metabolism disorders:* treatment should be avoided in patients with calcium metabolism disorders due to the risk of hypercalcaemia and hypercalciuria
- *Inflammatory psoriasis:* caution should be observed in patients with generalized pustular or erythrodermic psoriasis, due to the increased risk of hypercalcaemia and hypercalciuria as well as an increased risk of irritation (use should be suspended during any inflammatory flare of psoriasis

Common problems

- Vitamin D analogs are generally safe, but up to 25% of users will experience side effects, mostly local skin reactions including itching, erythema, a burning sensation, or dermatitis.

Treatment pearls

- Products are formulated as ointments (suitable for the body) as well as solutions or gels (e.g. for hair bearing areas including scalp)

- Calcipotriol is more effective than calcitriol and tacalcitol for the treatment of chronic plaque psoriasis, but is also more likely to cause irritation

- For psoriasis affecting 'sensitive areas' such the face and flexures, calcitriol may be more effective and better tolerated than calcipotriol

- The initial response to topical vitamin D and its analogs may be seen after 2–4 weeks; an evaluation after 4 weeks of treatment is recommended

- Vitamin D analogs are not effective for the treatment of nail psoriasis

- Patients should wash their hands thoroughly after use to prevent inadvertent transfer of the product to other areas of the body

- If other medications are applied to the skin, for example topical corticosteroids, these should be applied at a different time of day (e.g. one at night and one in the morning)

- Topical treatments, including vitamin D and its analogs, are important adjuncts to systemic agents (including 'biologics'); their concomitant use may allow a reduction in doses of systemic therapies

- Use of emollients containing urea or salicylic acid may help reduce plaque thickness and scale, improving the absorption and efficacy of subsequent applications of vitamin D analogs

This usually resolves after reducing the frequency of application, but treatment should be discontinued if it does not

- Tacalcitol and calcitriol are less likely to irritate than calcipotriol, which is more likely to cause irritation, especially in flexures

- There is a risk of hypercalcaemia and hypercalciuria if the dose exceeds recommended guidelines

- Less common adverse effects include contact dermatitis and increased photosensitivity to UVB phototherapy

Further reading

Jabbar-Lopez ZK, Wu K, Reynolds NJ. Newer agents for psoriasis in adults. BMJ 2014; 349:g4026.

Ortonne JP, Humbert P, Nicolas JF, et al. Intra-individual comparison of the cutaneous safety and efficacy of calcitriol 3 microg g(-1) ointment and calcipotriol 50 microg g(-1) ointment on chronic plaque psoriasis localized in facial, hairline, retroauricular or flexural areas. Br J Dermatol 2003; 148:326–333.

Tremezaygues L, Reichrath J. Vitamin D analogs in the treatment of psoriasis: Where are we standing and where will we be going? Dermatoendocrinology 2011; 3:180–186.

Systemic therapies

Acitretin

Dermatologic indications

- Psoriasis, pityriasis rubra pilaris, Darier's disease
- *Also used for:* Ichthyoses (lamellar ichthyosis, X-lined ichthyosis), palmoplantar keratodermas, hidradenitis suppurativa
- *Sometimes used for:* Chemoprevention of non-melanoma skin cancer in high-risk populations, pustular dermatoses, cutaneous lupus erythematosus, hypertrophic lichen planus, disseminated superficial actinic porokeratosis, cutaneous T-cell lymphoma

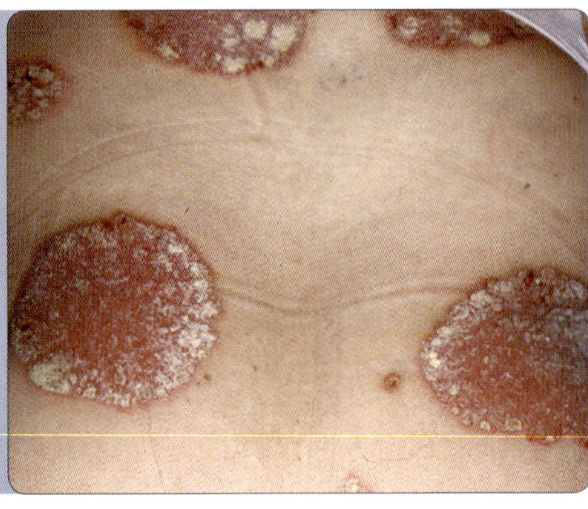

Figure 23.1 Psoriasis. Multiple pink plaques with silvery scales on the trunk.

Background

Acitretin is a second generation aromatic synthetic retinoid and an active metabolite of the closely-related agent etretinate.

It binds to retinoic acid receptors (RARs) which interact with specific target sequences in DNA to impact regulation of DNA transcription. This alteration of transcription leads to normalization of epidermal keratinocyte proliferation and differentiation.

Additionally, the release of inflammatory mediators such as leukotrienes and vascular endothelial growth factor are also down-regulated by acitretin. Finally, fibroblast growth and proliferation are down-regulated.

Dermatologic prescribing

- *Route:* oral
- *Oral dosing:* 10–50 mg once daily as a single dose. Treatment is often initiated at 25 mg once daily (generally 0.2–0.5 mg/kg/day), with dose adjustment based on efficacy and side-effect tolerability (up to 0.3–0.8 mg/kg/day). Tablets are available in 10 mg, 17.5 mg, and 25 mg doses
- Administration with meals enhances absorption
- Regular monitoring of complete blood count, renal function tests, liver function tests, serum glucose, and lipid panel are essential
- All women of reproductive age should be part of a pregnancy prevention program with regular screening while taking acitretin. Two forms of contraception are recommended during and for 3 years after treatment
- Individuals who develop multiple squamous cell carcinomas over a short period of time may benefit from the addition of low dose acitretin (10–25 mg/day). The benefit appears to be most pronounced in immunosuppressed individuals

(such as organ transplant recipients) or those with genetic predispositions to nonmelanoma skin cancer (such as individuals with xeroderma pigmentosum). The chemopreventive effect seems to be maintained only while the acitretin is continued. If acitretin is stopped, skin cancers typically develop. The use of acitretin in non-high risk groups for squamous cell carcinoma chemoprevention remains an area of investigation.

Cautions

- *Liver disease:* infectious hepatitis, advanced stage fatty liver, or excessive alcohol intake; acitretin is contraindicated with severe hepatic impairment
- *Renal disease:* partial renal excretion; acitretin is contraindicated with severe renal impairment
- *Hyperlipidemia:* elevates risk of hypertriglyceridemia, hypercholesterolemia
- *Medication interactions:* patients should be closely monitored if acitretin is used in conjunction with methotrexate (risk of liver injury) or tetracyclines (risk of intracranial hypertension). Patients should be counseled to avoid additional Vitamin A supplementation or combination use of other retinoids with acitretin
- *Pregnancy/lactation risk:* acitretin is a known teratogen. Acitretin is contraindicated in pregnancy and lactation as well as in women planning to conceive during therapy or within 3 years after completing treatment. Progestin-based oral contraceptives are not considered effective
- *Blood donation:* patients should not donate blood for 3 years after completing treatment to avoid possible exposure of acitretin-containing blood products to women of childbearing age

Common problems

- *Dermatologic:* cheilitis, xerostomia (up to 75% of patients), xerosis, paronychia, nail changes, alopecia

- *Hepatotoxicity:* elevated liver enzymes (up to 50% of patients), alkaline phosphatase, and serum bilirubin. Values are rarely more than three times the upper limit of normal. There have been rare reports of drug-induced hepatitis, which is an indication for drug discontinuation

- *Lipid abnormalities:* hypertriglyceridemia (up to 66% of patients), hypercholesterolemia, elevated serum glucose, decreased HDL cholesterol

- *Ocular:* xerophthalmia

- *Musculoskeletal:* increased creatine kinase, myalgias, arthralgias, spinal hyperostosis (seen with long-term treatment >2 years)

- *Nasal:* rhinitis, epistaxis

- *Gastrointestinal:* nausea, vomiting

- *Dose reduction:* doses <25 mg/day tend to have less pronounced side effects

Further reading

Menter A, Korman NJ, Elmets CA, et al. Guidelines of care for the management and treatment of psoriasis with traditional systemic agents. J Am Acad Dermatol 2009; 61:451–485.

Ormerod AD, Campalani E, Goodfield MJ; BAD Clinical Standards Unit. British Association of Dermatologists guidelines on the efficacy and use of acitretin in dermatology. Br J Dermatol 2010; 162:952–963.

Sarkar R, Chugh S, Garg VK. Acitretin in dermatology. Indian J Dermatol Venereol Leprol 2013; 79:759–771.

Treatment pearls

- The onset of action of acitretin may not be observed until 1–3 months after initiation

- Starting with low doses of acitretin and gradually dose-escalating over the course of 3 months may result in improved tolerability

- In patients with psoriasis, combination treatments of acitretin with topical agents (such as topical corticosteroids or vitamin D analogs) or additional treatment modalities (such as ultraviolet light alone or with psoralens) may be necessary for full disease clearance. Acitretin added to PUVA or UVB therapy may reduce the total number of ultraviolet treatment sessions necessary to achieve clearance

- Low doses (10 mg per day) of acitretin may be sufficient for chronic maintenance dosing in individuals with Darier's disease

- Consumption of acitretin with a fatty meal enhances its absorption

- Abstinence from alcohol while on acitretin can decrease reverse-esterification to etretinate and shorten the wash-out period to 3 months

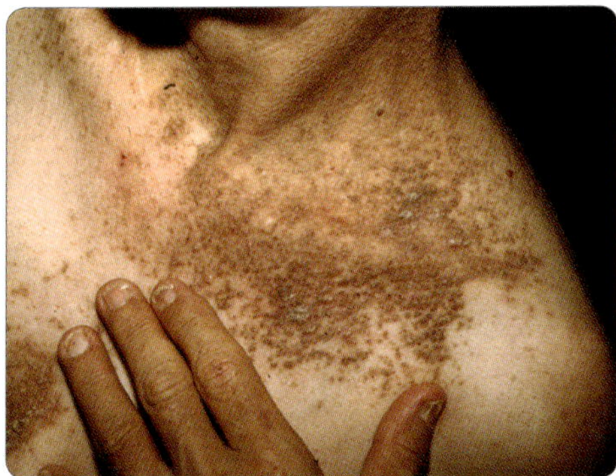

Figure 23.2 Darier's disease. Upper torso with tan-brown keratotic papules and fingernails demonstrating characteristic V-nicking and striping changes.

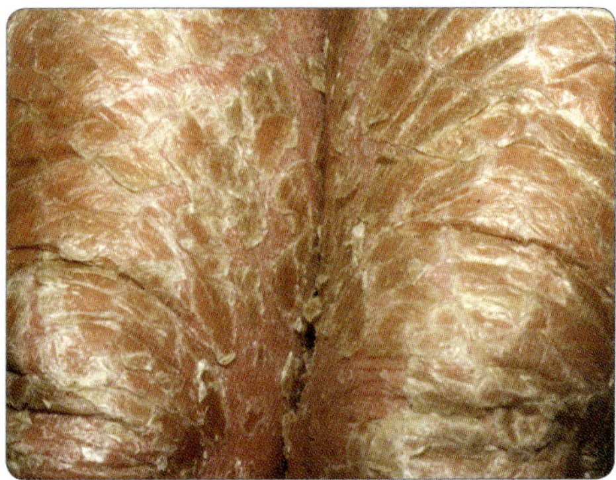

Figure 23.3 Lamellar ichthyosis. Diffuse adherent plate-like scale and underlying erythroderma.

Alitretinoin

Dermatologic indications

- Chronic severe hand eczema
- Kaposi's sarcoma
- *Also used for:* cutaneous T-cell lymphoma

Background

Alitretinoin is a first generation retinoid.

Its scientific name is 9-cis retinoic acid.

It binds to both retinoic acid receptors (RARs) and to retinoid X receptors (RXRs), which interact with specific target sequences in DNA to impact regulation of DNA transcription. This alteration of transcription leads to decreased proliferation of neoplastic cells in Kaposi's sarcoma.

The mechanism of action in chronic hand eczema is thought to be transcriptional alteration resulting in down-regulation of pro-inflammatory cytokines and normalization of keratinocyte proliferation.

Dermatologic prescribing

- *Route:* oral or topical
- *Oral dosing:* for treatment of chronic hand eczema: 10–30 mg once daily as a single dose. Available in 10 mg and 30 mg capsules. Lower doses are generally associated with fewer side effects
- Administration with meals enhances absorption of oral alitretinoin
- Regular (typically every 3 months) monitoring of complete blood count, renal function tests, liver function tests, serum glucose, thyroid function, and lipid panel are essential for individuals on oral alitretinoin
- All women require negative pregnancy tests before initiation, at baseline, and monthly while taking alitretinoin and for 1 month thereafter
- Two forms of contraception are required for women on alitretinoin and for 1 month thereafter
- *Topical dosing:* for treatment of Kaposi's sarcoma: twice daily application to skin lesions initially, up-titrated as tolerated based on side effects. Available in 0.1% topical gel formulation. Laboratory monitoring not required for topical use. Avoid in pregnant or lactating women

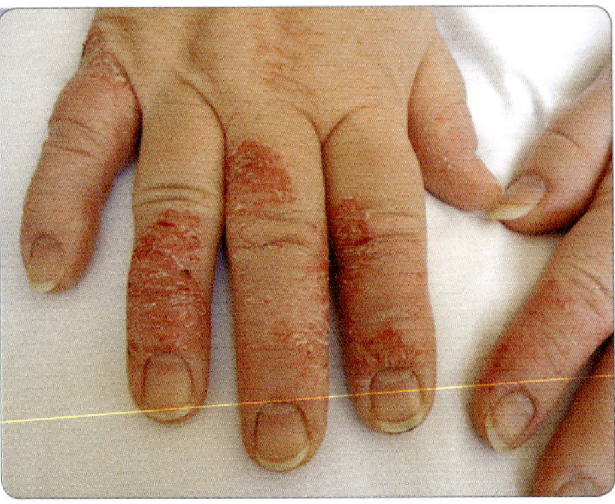

Figure 24.1 Chronic irritant dermatitis of the hands.

Cautions

- Oral alitretinoin
- *Liver disease:* infectious hepatitis, advanced stage fatty liver, or excessive alcohol intake; contraindicated with severe hepatic impairment
- *Renal disease:* partial renal excretion; contraindicated with severe renal impairment
- *Hyperlipidemia:* elevates risk of hypertriglyceridemia, hypercholesterolemia
- *Diabetes mellitus:* may elevate fasting serum glucose; close glucose monitoring
- *Medication interactions:* alitretinoin is a substrate of CYP3A4 and use should be monitored closely in individuals on CYP3A4 inducers or inhibitors. Co-administration of specific CYP3A4 inhibitors (conivaptan, fusidic acid, idelalisib, and stiripentol) should be avoided. Avoid using systemic alitretinoin with methotrexate (risk of liver injury) or tetracyclines (risk of benign intracranial hypertension). Alitretinoin decreases the efficacy of progestin-based oral contraceptives; these should not be used as a form of birth control during or after treatment. Patients must avoid additional Vitamin A supplementation or combination use of other retinoids
- Topical alitretinoin
- *DEET:* alitretinoin should not be used in combination with topical insect repellants containing diethyltoluamide (DEET) due to potential drug interaction
- *Pregnancy/lactation risk:* alitretinoin is a known teratogen. Both oral and topical alitretinoin are

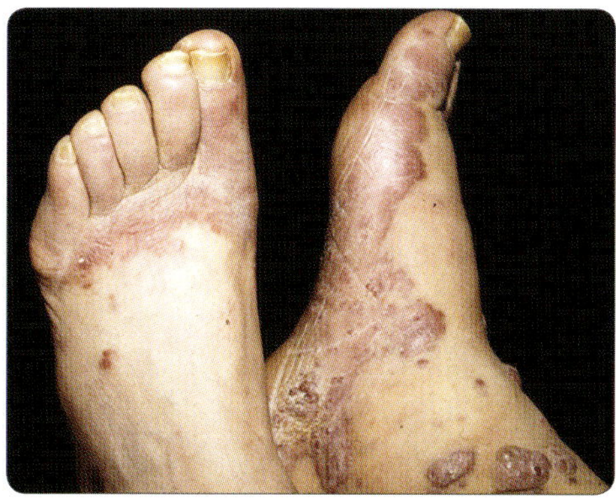

Figure 24.2 Kaposi's sarcoma. Purplish-red plaques and nodules on the bilateral lower extremities.

contraindicated in pregnancy and for 1 month thereafter as well as in lactation

- *Blood donation:* patients should not donate blood for 1 month after completing treatment to avoid possible exposure of alitretinoin-containing blood products to women of childbearing age

Common problems

- Oral alitretinoin
- *Neurologic:* headache (up to 20%)
- *Lipid abnormalities:* hypercholesterolemia (elevated LDL cholesterol), decreased HDL cholesterol, hypertriglyceridemia, elevated serum glucose
- *Dermatologic:* erythema, cheilitis, xerostomia, xerosis
- *Hepatotoxicity:* transient, reversible elevated liver enzymes, alkaline phosphatase, and serum bilirubin. Usually mild
- *Ocular:* xerophthalmia, conjunctivitis
- *Musculoskeletal:* increased creatine kinase, myalgias, arthralgias
- *Gastrointestinal:* nausea, vomiting
- *Dose reduction:* doses of 10 mg/day tend to have less pronounced side effects
- Topical alitretinoin
- *Dermatologic:* rash (up to 75% of patients), pruritus, pain/burning, or paresthesia at site of application. Increased local photosensitivity

Treatment pearls

- The half-life of oral alitretinoin is 10 hours
- Due to risk of teratogenicity, contraception is required during systemic treatment and for one month after completion of therapy
- Effective means of contraception include: tubal ligation, vasectomy, IUD, oral contraceptives, long-acting injected or implanted birth control, and barrier contraception
- Progestin-only pills should not be used for contraception while taking or for one month after completing alitretinoin due to decreased efficacy
- The most common side effect of oral alitretinoin use is headache, which is seen more commonly at 30 mg/day dosing than at 10 mg/day dosing
- Oral alitretinoin courses of up to 24 weeks may be necessary to achieve treatment response for chronic hand eczema
- Combination treatments of systemic alitretinoin with topical corticosteroids may be necessary for full disease clearance of chronic hand eczema
- Consumption of alitretinoin with a fatty meal will enhance absorption
- Topical alitretinoin gel should be avoided on mucosal surfaces to prevent irritation and systemic absorption

Further reading

Bodsworth NJ, Bloch M, Bower M, et al. Phase III vehicle-controlled, multi-centered study of topical alitretinoin gel 0.1% in cutaneous AIDS-related Kaposi's sarcoma. Am J Clin Dermatol 2001; 2:77–87.

Lynde C, Cambazard F, Ruzicka T, et al. Extended treatment with oral alitretinoin for patients with chronic hand eczema not fully responding to initial treatment. Clin Exp Dermatol 2012; 37:712–717.

Ruzicka T, Lynde CW, Jemec GB, et al. Efficacy and safety of oral alitretinoin (9-cis retinoic acid) in patients with severe chronic hand eczema refractory to topical corticosteroids: results of a randomized, double-blind, placebo-controlled, multicentre trial. Br J Dermatol 2008; 158:808–817.

Dermatologic indications

- *Cyproterone acetate:* moderate to severe acne (licensed), hirsutism (licensed), female pattern hair loss, seborrheic dermatitis, hidradenitis suppurativa in women of reproductive age

- *Spironolactone:* acne and/or hirsutism in women with evidence of androgen sensitivity, seborrheic dermatitis

- *Finasteride:* androgenetic alopecia (licensed) in men, androgenetic alopecia in women

Background

Circulating androgen sex hormones regulate sebum production which is associated with acne.

In genetically prone individuals, androgens induce some hair follicles to undergo miniaturization. In males this classically results in the characteristic pattern of androgenetic alopecia (syn. androgenic alopecia, male pattern baldness) showing frontal hair margin recession and occipital thinning. In women, excess androgens are associated with hirsuitism, acne and androgenetic alopecia (female pattern hair loss).

Cyproterone acetate

- Usually taken combined with ethinylestradiol (combined oral contraceptive: co-cyprindiol)
- Acts as anti-androgen:
- Suppression of luteinizing hormone
- Elevation of sex hormone-binding globulin (reducing bioavailability)
- Inhibition of conversion of free testosterone to dihydrotestosterone in skin and hair follicles

Spironolactone

- Aldosterone antagonist
- Reduces adrenal androgen production
- Blocks androgen receptors

Finasteride

- 5α-reductase inhibitor targeting type II/III isoenzymes
- Prevents conversion of testosterone to dihydrotestosterone, resulting in reduction of local and systemic androgen effects
- Acts on hair follicles, reversing hair miniaturization

Dermatologic prescribing

Co-cyprindiol

- Cyproterone acetate 2 mg with ethinylestradiol 35 µg

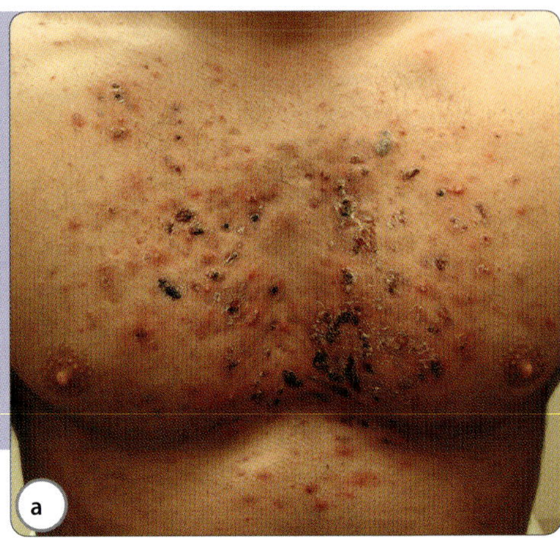

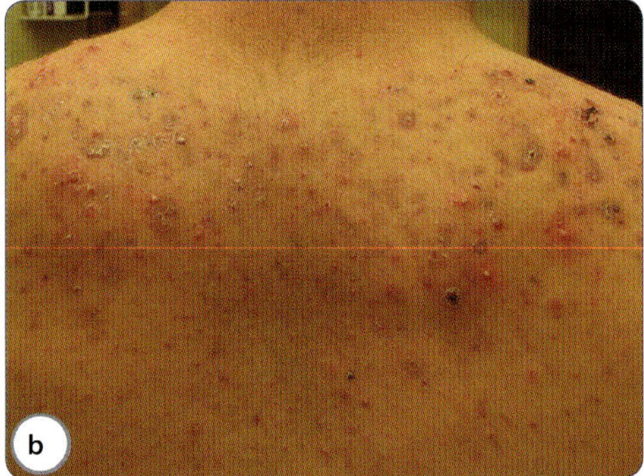

Figure 25.1 Inflammatory, scarring acne. (a) Front, (b) back.

- One tablet daily starting on day 1 of the menstrual cycle for 21 days, then withheld for 7 days (for withdrawal bleeding) before repeating

Spironolactone

- 25–200 mg per day divided in 1–2 doses
- Healthy young women: monitoring is not usually necessary
- Concomitant use of nephrotoxic medication, significant renal or cardiac impairment
- Potassium and creatinine should be monitored 1 week after initiation and after any dose increase, monthly for first 3 months, then every 3 months for 1 year and then every 6 months). The dose should be reduced or treatment discontinued if hyperkalemia occurs

Finasteride

- 1 mg/day (no significant difference in efficacy between this dose and 5 mg/day)

Cautions

- All women require contraception while being treated with spironolactone or finasteride as these medications will feminize a male fetus. Co-cyprindiol is a hormone contraceptive. Therefore it should not be used with other hormone contraceptives

Co-cyprindiol

- Contraindications are the same as for a combined oral contraceptive pill. Prior consideration of venous thromboembolism risk is important. Risk factors, including smoking, should be assessed in all patients

Finasteride

- Reduces prostate specific antigen (PSA) levels, and may potentially delay a diagnosis of prostate cancer. Practitioners should consider checking PSA levels before treatment, with regular monitoring while on treatment in those aged over 45 years, doubling the levels to account for the effect of finasteride
- Breast cancer has been reported in males taking finasteride. Patients should be informed and advised of the signs for which to monitor
- Hypersensitivity reactions can occur

Spironolactone

- Use in the setting of men should be avoided due to the risk of feminization
- Use in acute or severe renal impairment, hyperkalemia, and Addison's disease should also be avoided
- Use in pregnancy should be avoided due to the potential feminization of the male fetus. Contraception should be used
- The use of other drugs that might reduce renal function and increase the risk of hyperkalemia (e.g. ACE inhibitors, angiotensin II receptor antagonists, and NSAIDs) should be employed with caution
- Potentially serious interactions can occur if used with lithium, cyclosporine, tacrolimus, and digoxin
- Patients should be informed of the theoretical risk of malignancy (shown to be carcinogenic in rodents)

Common problems

Co-cyprindiol

- Headaches, breast tenderness, mood change, weight gain, nausea, and abdominal pain

Finasteride

- Men
- Increased risk of erectile dysfunction (1 in 80 patients)
- Discuss reports of decreased libido and infertility, but stress that no causal link has been found

Treatment pearls

- Combination with weight loss in overweight patients provides added improvement in anti-androgen effects

Finasteride

- There is limited evidence for its use in androgenetic alopecia in women
- Pre-treatment photographs of the scalp can help with monitoring response to therapy
- Patients can expect a 30% improvement in hair loss when used long-term
- The treatment response at 6 months should be reviewed, though a response may not be evident until 1 year of treatment in some patients
- Combining the use of finasteride with topical minoxidil is more effective than either treatment alone

Spironolactone

- Gradual dose titration upwards to therapeutic effect is less likely to cause side effects

Co-cyprindiol

- Cyproterone acetate when combined with ethinylestradiol is an effective contraception in patients requiring it for the above conditions, but it should not be used solely for contraceptive purposes
- Can be used in combination with systemic antibiotics or topical therapies for acne
- May be used in combination with hair removal techniques (shaving, waxing, plucking, bleaching, electrolysis, or laser therapy) for hirsutism

- Women
- Increased libido and breast tenderness, which may resolve with continued use

Spironolactone

- Postural hypotension, breast tenderness, menstrual irregularities

Further reading

Arowojolu AO, Gallo MF, Lopez LM, Grimes DA. Combined oral contraceptive pills for treatment of acne. Cochrane Database of Systematic Reviews 2012; 7: CD004425.

Mella JM, Perret MC, Manzotti M, et al. Efficacy and safety of finasteride therapy for androgenetic alopecia. A systematic review. Arch Dermatol 2010; 146: 1141–1150.

Nast A, Dréno B, Bettoli V, et al. European evidence-based (S3) guidelines for the treatment of acne. J Eur Acad Dermatol Venereol 2012; 26:1–29.

Antibiotics for acne

Dermatologic indications

- Oral antibiotics as part of a treatment regimen are indicated for moderate to severe facial acne and/or extensive truncal acne

Background

Acne is the most common inflammatory dermatosis seen worldwide. It frequently has a prolonged course and varies in severity and extent.

Clinical presentation includes non-inflammatory (blackheads and whiteheads) and/or inflammatory (papules, pustules, and nodules) most commonly distributed over the face and/or trunk. Excessive sebum production is frequent. Physical and emotional scarring is common and more likely if treatment is delayed.

The pathophysiology of acne involves defects in sebum synthesis and is associated with hyperkeratinization in the upper part of the pilosebaceous follicle. Multiplication of *Propionibacterium acnes* (*P. acnes*) within the blocked follicles leads to inflammation involving both the adaptive and innate immune responses. Systemic antibiotics have been the cornerstone of acne management strategies for over 50 years. In vitro but not in vivo data suggest they may work not only by reducing the burden of of *P. acnes*, but also via direct anti-inflammatory/immunomodulatory effects on cells of the immune system.

Increasing concerns regarding antibiotic resistance are yet to impact prescribing for acne, but may do so in the future.

Dermatologic prescribing

- *Tetracyclines:* (oxytetracycline, doxycycline, lymecycline, minocycline) are the antibiotics of choice for acne. There is insufficient evidence to support one agent or dose over another. **Table 26.1** provides information on the dosage regimens commonly adopted

- Second generation tetracyclines (lymecycline and doxycycline) may improve compliance due to once daily dosing. These are often used in preference to minocycline which can have more serious adverse effects and is not as cost effective

- *Macrolides:* (erythromycin, clindamycin, azithromycin) for acne have increasingly fallen out of favor due to the emergence of antibiotic-resistant strains of *P. acnes* and evidence suggesting tetracycline is equivalent or superior in efficacy to erythromycin

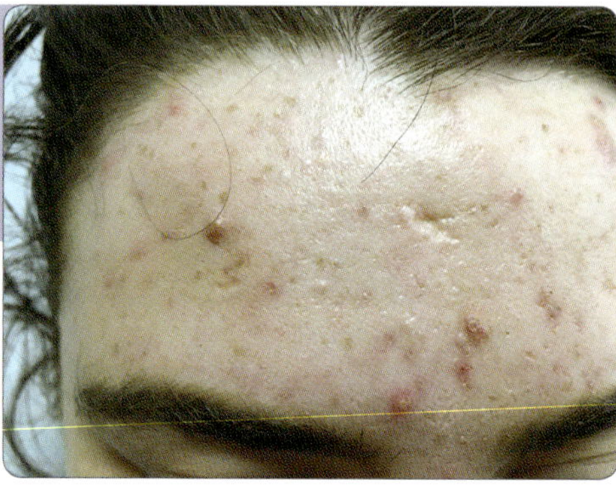

Figure 26.1 Acne on the forehead with comedones, inflammatory papules and ice pick scarring.

- When oral antibiotics are clinically justified, courses should be no longer than required to achieve good control, for most this will be 3–4 months. Response should be at least 50% improvement versus baseline. Experts recommend that clinical response to oral antibiotics be reviewed after 6–8 weeks, based on clinical trial evidence showing that if a patient is going to respond, improvement will be apparent after this period. Following a good response, treatment should be stopped, with maintenance topical treatment continued until complete acne resolution

- Co-prescribing of benzoyl peroxide is recommended as evidence suggests that this may reduce the development of antibiotic resistance. Co-prescribing of topical retinoids will expedite improvement and reduce exposure to antibiotics. Removing the follicular occlusion is essential in producing long-term resolution of acne

Common problems

- All oral antibiotics for acne can produce adverse effects (**Table 26.1**)

- Oral antibiotics for acne drive resistance in targeted and non-targeted bacteria at multiple body sites. The presence of antibiotic-resistant *P. acnes* may lead to reduced response to antibiotics

Further reading

Nast A, Dréno B, Bettoli V, et al. European evidence-based (S3) guidelines for the treatment of acne. J Eur Acad Dermatol Venereol 2012; 26:1–29.

National Institute for Health and Care Excellence. NICE Clinical Knowledge Summaries: Acne Vulgaris. London: NICE, 2014.

Thiboutot D, Gollnick, H, Bettoli V, et al. New insights into the management of acne: an update from the Global Alliance to Improve Outcomes in Acne group. J Am Acad Dermatol 2009; 60:S1–S50.

Table 26.1 Dosage and adverse effects of systemic antibiotics used for acne

Antibiotics for acne	Dosage regimens	Adverse effects
Oxytetracycline	500 mg twice daily taken half an hour before food and not with milk (this can compromise absorption of the medication)	Common: gastrointestinal upset Rare: onycholysis, photosensitivity, benign intracranial hypertension
Lymecycline (not available in the US)	408–816 mg daily, equivalent to tetracycline	Similar to oxytetracycline but tolerated better and can be taken with food
Doxycycline	100 mg once- or twice-daily	Similar to oxytetracycline Photosensitivity (dose-dependent)
Minocycline	100 mg once- or twice-daily	Pigmentary changes Rare but serious: vertigo, headaches and dizziness associated with benign intracranial hypertension, autoimmune hepatitis/lupus erythematosus-like syndrome
Erythromycin	500 mg twice daily	Common: gastrointestinal upset, nausea, diarrhea
Trimethoprim	200–300 mg twice daily	Morbilliform drug eruption, severe drug eruptions Rare: hepatic/renal toxicity/agranulocytosis

Treatment pearls

- ■ Antibiotic prescribing policies aimed at achieving optimal therapeutic response while avoiding antibiotic resistance suggest:
- ● Restricting the duration of antibiotics (typically 3–6 months average duration)
- ● Avoid combinations of different oral and topical antibiotics and regular switching of antibiotics
- ● Assess clinical efficacy after 6–8 weeks and stop ineffective courses
- ● Use alternative treatments and transfer antibiotic-treated patients onto antibiotic-free maintenance regimens as soon as controlled
- ● Use concomitant benzoyl peroxide which reduces the emergence of antibiotic resistant strains of *P. acnes*
- ● Use concomitant topical retinoids to expedite response and reduce exposure to antibiotics
- ● Refer patients with recalcitrant acne to secondary care early
- ■ Despite reports of efficacy in acne, the use of azithromycin, trimethoprim, and other antibiotics including cephalosporins and flourquinolones should be minimized as they are commonly used to treat a variety of systemic infections
- ■ Oral clindamycin is effective in acne, but adverse effects, including diarrhea, seen in 5–20% of cases, and potential pseudomembranous colitis from overgrowth of *Clostridium difficile,* has discouraged use
- ■ Concern that combined oral contraceptive (COC) efficacy may be impaired when used in conjunction with systemic antibiotics is based on the hypothesis that broad-spectrum antibiotics reduce bacterial flora in the gut and may interfere with estrogen absorption. Pharmacokinetic studies demonstrate that serum levels of estrogen are unaffected by tetracycline and doxycycline. The failure rate of COCs when used with tetracycline resulting in pregnancy is reported as 1.2–1.4 pregnancies per 100 woman-years of COC use, which is no greater than their background failure rate. Importantly, the only antibiotic which has been shown to reduce COC efficacy is rifampicin
- ■ Tetracyclines should not be used in conjunction with oral isotretinoin due to risk of benign intracranial hypertension
- ■ If antibiotic therapy is required in pregnancy, oral erythromycin is deemed to be safe
- ■ Erythromycin remains the preferred option in children (8–12 years, depending on country) as tetracylines are contraindicated due to potential musculoskeletal problems and discoloration of permanent teeth

Antibiotics for skin infections

Dermatologic indications

- Skin infections such as cellulitis, erysipelas and folliculitis
- Inflammatory skin conditions with a presumed bacterial trigger or bacterial colonization such as folliculitis decalvans and hidradenitis suppurativa

Background

Cellulitis

- Cellulitis is a common bacterial infection of the lower dermis and subcutaneous tissue presenting with erythema, swelling, warmth, and pain. The skin may be eroded, ulcerated, or blistered. It is usually caused by *Streptococcus pyogenes* or *Staphylococcus aureus*

- In addition to oral or parenteral antibiotics, treatment includes elevation of any affected limb and analgesia

- Compared with inpatient care, the mean duration of treatment with parenteral antibiotics at home (outpatient parenteral antibiotic treatment) has been shown to be similar, but is almost half the cost. Additionally, patient and care-giver satisfaction with home-based care is high

- Antibiotics for patients with lymphedema should be continued until all signs of acute inflammation have resolved. This may mean taking antibiotics for 1–2 months, and the course of antibiotics should be continued for no less than 14 days from the time a definite clinical response is observed

Erysipelas

- Erysipelas is a superficial infection affecting the upper layers of the skin. The borders are often raised, sharply demarcated, and advancing, with rapid enlargement over 3–6 days. The face and legs are the most commonly involved sites

- On the face, the source of bacteria is usually the nasopharynx. Most infections are caused by group A streptococci

Erythrasma

- Erythrasma presents as a pink or brown, slowly enlarging, patch of skin with fine scale, which may be pruritic. It is caused by *Corynebacterium minutissimum,* a component of normal skin flora, which often coexists with dermatophytes or *Candida albicans*. It is particularly prevalent in diabetics and those living in warm climates. It may become widespread and invasive in

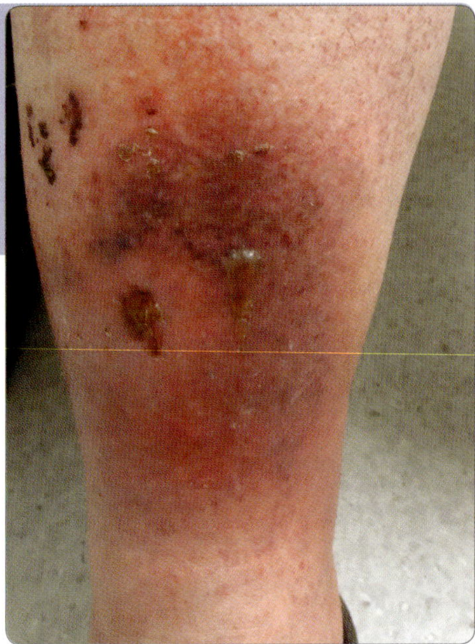

Figure 27.1 Cellulitis on the lower leg with blistering and superficial erosions.

immunocompromised individuals, allowing abscess formation, cellulitis, and endocarditis to occur

- A diagnosis is made by examining the skin with a Wood's light and observing the characteristic coral-pink fluorescence which is caused by release of porphyrins by the bacteria. Results may be negative if the patient has bathed prior to presentation. The diagnosis can be confirmed by taking swabs for bacterial culture and/or skin scrapings for microscopy and culture

- Treatment of erythrasma can be with topical antibiotics such as fusidic acid cream, clindamycin solution, erythromycin gel, or Whitfield's (compound benzoic acid) ointment. Oral antibiotics such as erythromycin or tetracyclines are also used. Antibacterial soap can be used to prevent recurrence

Folliculitis

- Folliculitis is characterized by papules and pustules on an erythematous base that are usually pierced by a central hair. It is often associated with pruritus

- The most commonly affected sites are the face, scalp, thighs, axillae, and inguinal area. Folliculitis is usually caused by *S. aureus* infection, and patients suffering repeated episodes should

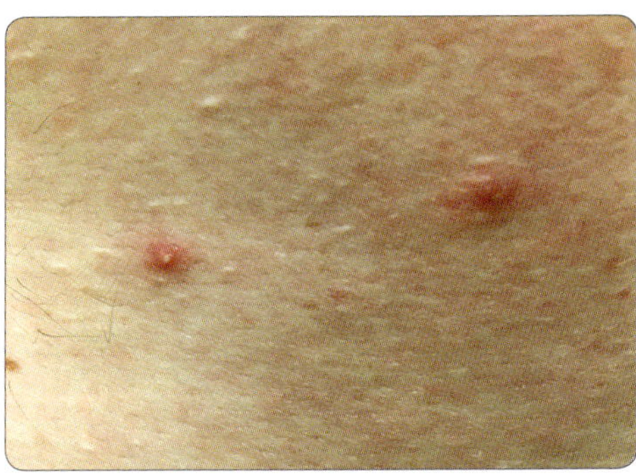

Figure 27.2 Folliculitis affecting the lower back.

be swabbed to exclude nasal Staphylococcal carriage. For recurrent uncomplicated superficial folliculitis, use of topical antibacterial agents may be all that is required. For persistent or deep lesions, oral antibiotics with adequate coverage of *S. aureus* should be prescribed

Dermatologic prescribing

The choice of antibiotics should be determined by bacterial culture results with sensitivities as well as by patient allergies.

Treatment duration is usually for 7 days initially. Antibiotics used for common skin infections in dermatology include:

- Flucloxacillin 250–500 mg four times daily
- Penicillin V 500 mg four times daily
- Penicillin V for prophylaxis of lower limb cellulitis 250 mg twice daily
- Cephalexin 250–500 mg four times daily
- Erythromycin 250–500 mg four times daily
- Clindamycin 150–300 mg four times daily
- Linezolid 600 mg twice daily (needs monitoring)

Common problems

- Always check for allergies to antibiotics
- Penicillin is a common cause of drug eruptions, including morbilliform drug eruptions, but also drug reaction with eosinophilia and systemic symptoms (DRESS) and acute generalized exanthematous pustulosis (AGEP)
- Clindamycin can cause *C. difficile* diarrhea
- For moderate skin and soft tissue infections with MSSA use either: flucloxacillin 500 mg four times a day or clindamycin 450 mg four times a day
- Methicillin resistant *Staphylococcus aureus* (MRSA)
- The type of infections caused by MRSA are the same as those caused by other staphylococcal organisms, i.e. MRSA is not more virulent or infectious than other staphylococcal species
- MRSA occurs worldwide and is more prevalent in institutional settings. The most important reservoir of infection is patients who may have colonization of the nostrils, groin, axillae, and/or wounds. Colonized patients have a 30–60% risk of developing infection, presumably due to factors related to their intercurrent illness. In the UK, MRSA bacteremia is a recognized healthcare associated infection (HCAI) and part of mandatory surveillance and reporting
- The antibiotic of choice should be determined by microbiologic sensitivities but is typically intravenous glycopeptides (vancomycin or teicoplanin) for inpatients. Oral clindamycin or doxycycline may be used in minor soft tissue infections in the outpatient setting. Co-trimoxazole is also effective against staphylococcal skin infections.
- Newer antibiotics such as linezolid, daptomycin, quinupristin/dalfopristin, tigecycline and ceftaroline may be used if infections fail to respond to glycopeptides
- Healthcare workers who are colonized with MRSA rarely develop infection. As treatment of MRSA infection is difficult, prevention of infection is important
- To reduce persistent MRSA carriage, underlying skin conditions (such as eczema) should be treated, invasive devices should be removed and/or replaced, and any loss of skin integrity should be managed
- A typical eradication regimen may include intranasal 2% mupirocin ointment three times daily for 5 days and 4% chlorhexidine gluconate body-wash/shampoo, 7.5% povidone iodine, or 2% triclosan daily for 5 days. To establish that MRSA eradication has been successful, three screens 1 week apart are performed. Clinicians should refer to their local MRSA screening/treatment policies for up-to-date guidance
- Clinical practice guidelines for the treatment of MRSA infections in adults and children have been published by the Infectious Diseases Society of America
- Panton-Valentine leukocidin (PVL)
- PVL is a toxin produced by some strains of *S. aureus*. (PVL-SA) and predominantly causes skin and soft tissue infections but can also cause invasive infections
- The cutaneous manifestations of PVL-SA infection, which are often recurrent, include boils, carbuncles, folliculitis, cellulitis, and

purulent eyelid infections. Pain and erythema out of proportion to the severity of infection and tissue necrosis can be indicators of PVL-SA infection. PVL-SA should also be suspected if there is clustering of infections within a social or household group. Risk factors for infection include compromised skin integrity, skin to skin contact, and sharing of contaminated items such as towels, toothbrushes etc.

- When PVL-MRSA is suspected and hospital admission is not warranted use: rifampicin 300 mg twice daily + doxycycline (100 mg twice daily – not for children <12 years of age) or rifampicin 300 mg twice daily + fusidic acid 500 mg three times a day or rifampicin 300 mg twice daily + trimethoprim 200 mg twice daily or clindamycin 450 mg four times a day. Treatment should last 5–7 days

- For severe infections where PVL-SA (MSSA or MRSA) is suspected, parenteral vancomycin, teicoplanin, daptomycin or linezolid have been used. Tigecycline may also offer broader polymicrobial coverage

- Topical decolonization should be offered to all primary cases but is important to remember that suppression of PVL is ineffective if the skin lesions remain unhealed. Chlorhexidine 4% body wash/shampoo or triclosan 1–2% should be used daily as liquid soap when bathing for 5 days and as a shampoo on days 1, 3 and 5. Mupirocin ointment should be applied three times daily for 5 days to the inner surface of each nostril

Treatment pearls

- Whenever possible, the presence and sensitivity of bacterial infection should be established by taking bacterial swabs for culture and sensitivity

- If the practitioner is unsure about which antibiotic to use, they should consult their microbiology service

- Minor skin and soft tissue infections (SSTIs) will usually respond to topical antibiotic treatment unless the patient is immunocompromised, an infant, or deteriorating clinically. The optimal treatment for abscesses is incision and drainage. Moderate SSTIs including cellulitis and larger abscesses (especially those >5 cm) should be treated with oral anti-staphylococcal antibiotics in addition to incision and drainage in the case of abscesses

- In cases of lower limb cellulitis, an attempt to identify the cause and any predisposing factors should always be made. Many patients have co-existing tinea pedis leading to skin breaks allowing bacteria entry into the skin. Concomitant tinea pedis should be treated

- There are now high quality data demonstrating that prophylactic penicillin V (250 mg twice daily) can prevent further episodes in patients who have recurrent lower leg cellulitis

- If folliculitis is not responding to standard antibiotics, the following should be considered:

- Tinea infection: Tinea faciei (tinea barbae in men) may be caused by a zoophilic dermatophyte and is often seen in farm workers

- Gram-negative folliculitis, which occurs in patients on long-term antibiotic therapy and results from overgrowth of Gram-negative organisms at the expense of normal skin flora

- Pseudomonal folliculitis, which appears up to 48 hours after exposure to contaminated water or wet suits with clinical signs concentrated in areas occluded by swimwear. Hot tub folliculits is often due to pseudomonal infection

- Pityrosporum folliculitis, presents as intensely pruritic uniform papules on the back, chest, and shoulders and is due to infection with *Malassezia furfur*

- Other causes of folliculitis include overgrowth of demodex mites; infection with herpes simplex or varicella zoster virus; acute generalized exanthematous pustulosis; DRESS; folliculitis secondary to EGFR therapy; and Ofuji disease (eosinophilic folliculitis). A different form of eosinophilic folliculitis may also occur after antiretroviral therapy

Further reading

British Lymphology Society. Consensus Document on the Management of Cellulitis in Lymphoedema. London: British Lymphology Society and the Lymphoedema Support Network, 2016

Chapman AL, Dixon S, Andrews D, et al. Clinical efficacy and cost-effectiveness of outpatient parenteral antibiotic therapy (OPAT): a UK perspective. J Antimicrob Chemother 2009; 64:1316–1324.

Health Protection Agency. Guidance on the diagnosis and management of PVL-associated *Staphylococcus aureus* infections (PVL-SA) in England, 2nd Edition. London: Health Protection Agency, 2008.

Infectious Diseases Society of America. Clinical Practice Guidelines by the Infectious Diseases Society of America for the treatment of methicillin-resistant *Staphylococcus aureus* infections in adults and children. Arlington: Infectious Diseases Society of America, 2011.

Mason JM, Thomas KS, Crook AM, et al Prophylactic antibiotics to prevent cellulitis of the leg: economic analysis of the PATCH I & II trials. PLoS One 2014; 9:e82694.

Phoenix G, Das S, Joshi M. Diagnosis and management of cellulitis. BMJ 2012; 345:e4955.

Dermatologic indications

- Skin, nail, and hair infections due to dermatophytes (tinea), yeasts (e.g. *Candida* species), or molds, as well as mucosal candidiasis (fluconazole, nystatin, itraconazole)

- Some systemic mycoses (fluconazole and itraconazole only). Griseofulvin is only licensed for dermatophyte infections

- Widespread tinea pedis and tinea corporis, tinea capitis, onychomycosis, tinea (pityriasis) versicolor, oral and vulvovaginal candidiasis

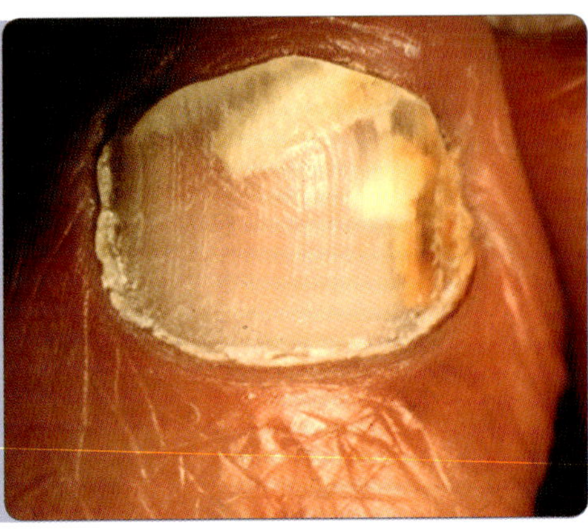

Figure 28.1 Onychomycosis due to *T. rubrum*. The streaks or dermatophytomas on the lateral nail are a clue to the fact that this patient's infection may respond poorly to treatment.

Background

Fungal infections of the skin such as tinea (dermatophyte infection) are usually itchy and may cover large areas; a raised margin can usually be identified. Other keratinized sites, e.g. hair, nails, may also be involved.

Some tinea infections, particularly those caused by fungi of animal origin, are usually inflamed and/or pustular. Many tinea infections of human origin show a striking lack of inflammation.

Tinea capitis, fungal infection of the scalp, presents with areas of scalp scaling and focal hair loss

Onychomycosis or fungal nail infection is usually caused by dermatophytes, but mold or *Candida* is sometimes implicated. *Candida* can also infect the nail folds causing chronic paronychia.

Oral treatment is used where the fungal infection is very extensive or chronic (e.g. *Candida* on mucosal surfaces) or when it involves hair or nails.

Some oral antifungals are also effective for both subcutaneous and systemic fungal infections such as mycetoma or histoplasmosis.

Terbinafine is very effective (fungicidal) against dermatophyte infections but ineffective orally against *Candida* and *Malassezia*.

Triazoles (e.g. itraconazole and fluconazole) are effective (fungistatic) against most *Candida* and *Malassezia* spp. (yeasts) as well as dermatophyte infections. Some *Candida* species (e.g. *C. glabrata* in vulvovaginal infections may be resistant to fluconazole.

Griseofulvin is used (second-line) for dermatophyte infections of the hair and, less commonly, the nails. It is often used first-line in children for tinea capitis.

Nystatin is an oral, non-absorbed medication for oral candidiasis (thrush).

Dermatologic prescribing

- Oral terbinafine 250 mg is usually prescribed once daily for 1–2 weeks for extensive dermatophyte infections, 4–6 weeks for tinea capitis; 6 weeks for fingernail and 12 weeks for toenail onychomycosis. Occasionally longer treatment times are required for nail infections

- Oral itraconazole 100 mg is usually prescribed daily for 2–4 weeks for extensive tinea corporis or cruris. It is typically given as 200 mg twice daily for a week each month for 2 months for fingernail and 3 months for toenail onychomycosis (pulsed therapy)

- Oral fluconazole can be given daily at 100 mg for oral and vulvovaginal infections for 7–14 days or as a single 200 mg dose for vulvovaginal candidiasis. It is also used in a weekly pulse dose of 100–400 mg for tinea capitis or onychomycosis

- The usual dose of griseofulvin is 500–1000 mg daily for 4–6 weeks for extensive tinea cruris or corporis and for up to 12 months for onychomycosis

- Combinations of terbinafine or itraconazole with topical nail preparations such as amorolfine or ciclopirox may be used for nail infections involving the entire nail plate

Common problems

- When treating extensive dermatophyte infections, relapse is common. This is seldom due to drug resistance

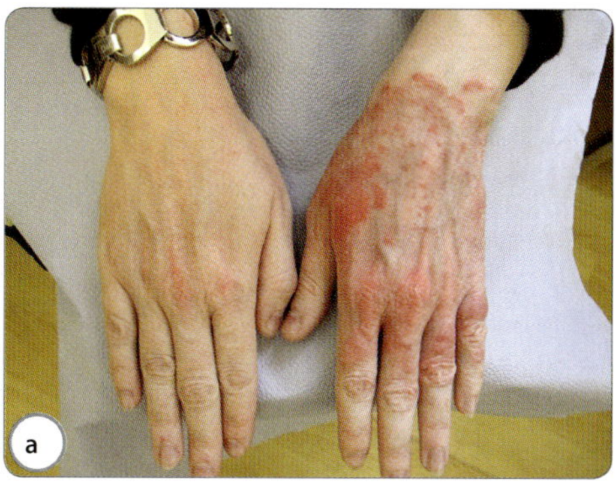

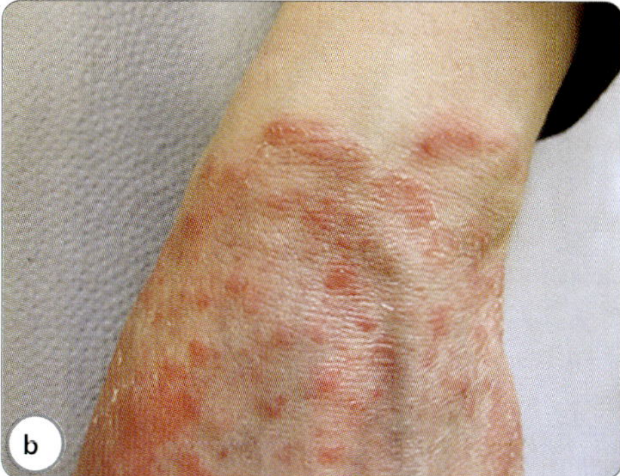

Figure 28.2 Both hands (a) and close up of left hand (b), showing a unilateral, scaly dermatitis on the dorsum of the left hand. A clearly defined, scaly margin and occasional pustule formation are hallmarks of tinea.

- Failure of treatment of onychomycosis occurs in 20–40% of those receiving treatment. Reasons include poor compliance, co-administration of drugs which affect absorption (e.g. rifampicin with itraconazole), or the presence of nail plate reservoirs of infection called streaks or dermatophytomas, which are often best removed surgically

- Confirmation of clinical diagnosis with mycologic sampling is recommended before oral therapy is commenced. Adequate samples of nail material should include as much nail and subungual debris as possible

- Terbinafine, itraconazole, and fluconazole produce similar adverse effects such as nausea and headache. Rare side effects include liver dysfunction and toxic epidermal necrolysis;

Treatment pearls

- If treating *Candida* paronychia with fluconazole or itraconazole, a strong topical steroid should be applied to the swollen nail fold for 2–3 weeks

- When considering oral antifungals, consider drug-drug interactions, which are most notably seen with itraconazole, but also with other agents

- Terbinafine is more active than azoles or griseofulvin for tinea capitis caused by *Trichophyton* species. The opposite is true for infections caused by *Microsporum* species

- Resistance of dermatophytes to oral antifungals is rare, but *Candida* species, even *C. albicans*, can become resistant to fluconazole when this drug is used over a long period in immunosuppressed patients

- Nystatin is seldom effective against oral candidiasis in immunosuppressed patients

- In patients who are immunosuppressed (e.g. those with HIV/AIDS), the normal daily dose of most oral antifungals can be doubled. Treatment duration is also longer

- Non-dermatophyte molds are more frequently found in nails and are usually resistant to standard treatment. Partial removal of the nail plate using 40% urea may be helpful in these cases

terbinafine and griseofulvin may cause dysgeusia/loss of taste. Griseofulvin may rarely cause leukopenia. Modification of dosing is necessary in patients with renal impairment

Further reading

de Sá DC, Lamas AP, Tosti A. Oral therapy for onychomycosis: an evidence-based review. Am J Clin Dermatol 2014; 15:17–36.

Eisman S, Sinclair R. Fungal nail infection: diagnosis and management. BMJ 2014; 348: g1800.

González U, Seaton T, Bergus G, et al. Systemic antifungal therapy for tinea capitis in children. Cochrane Database Syst Rev 2007; CD004685.

Antihistamines, sodium cromoglicate and leukotriene receptor antagonists

Dermatologic indications

- *Oral antihistamines:* urticaria, arthropod bites and stings, various cutaneous eruptions associated with pruritus, anaphylaxis, histaminergic (but not hereditary) angioedema

- *Oral sodium cromoglicate (Nalcrom):* bowel symptoms in systemic mastocytosis

- *Leukotriene receptor antagonists (LTRA):* chronic urticaria as an adjunct to other therapies, symptom control in systemic mastocytosis.

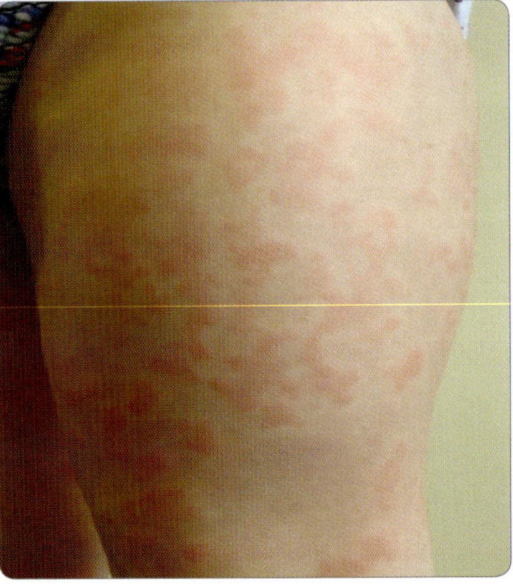

Figure 29.1 Widespread urticaria on the leg of a child.

Background

Urticaria ('hives') is characterized by raised wheals in the skin which are typically itchy and short-lived (last <24 hours). Wheals can be round, polycyclic or annular and may be <1cm or cover large areas of skin. Acute urticaria (lasting <6 weeks) may represent allergic IgE mediated degranulation of mast cells, and the potential for anaphylaxis needs to be considered. Most cases of chronic urticaria (lasting >6 weeks) are not allergic and often no cause is identified. Both allergic and non-allergic urticaria are mediated by degranulation of mast cells in the superficial dermis (wheals) or deep dermis (angiodema), and the principal active molecule is histamine. Antihistamines block the effect of histamine on its receptors (H1-4) but do not stabilize the mast cell.

First generation antihistamines readily cross the blood brain barrier and cause sedation, whereas newer antihistamines are non-sedating (**Table 29.1**).

Oral sodium cromoglycate stabilizes mast cells, but is not absorbed from the gut so is primarily used for bowel symptoms in systemic mastocytosis.

Cysteinyl leukotrienes are pro-inflammatory mediators synthesized at the time of mast cell degranulation, which can be blocked by leukotriene receptor antagonists, such as montelukast and zafirlukast.

Urticaria treatment pearls

- International consensus guidelines recommend that non-sedating antihistamines may be used in up to fourfold the licensed dosages for the treatment of chronic urticaria. Patients with urticaria who fail to respond to antihistamine therapy are often underdosed

- Evidence does not support switching antihistamines to achieve greater therapeutic effect

- The efficacy of antihistamines is greater when taken regularly rather than as needed

- Non-sedating H1 antihistamines are often used in combination with sedating H1 and H2 antihistamines in cases of chronic or refractory urticaria

- In patients with atopic dermatitis (atopic eczema), sedating antihistamines may be useful to aid sleep at night and help break the itch-scratch cycle. Non-sedating antihistamines may help reduce oral or aero-allergen triggered histamine flares

- Grapefruit and orange juice reduce blood levels of fexofenadine, while grapefruit juice increases levels of rupatadine

- Loratadine and cetirizine are the preferred options for antihistamine use in pregnancy if the benefits of treatment are thought to outweigh any risks

- LTRAs may be used in combination with non-sedating H1 antihistamines for symptomatic relief of chronic urticaria

Table 29.1 Antihistamine dosages for management of chronic urticaria

Generic name	Children under 12 years of age	Adults and children 12–18 years of age (>40 kg)
Non- or low-sedating antihistamines		
Acrivastine	Unlicensed	8 mg three times daily
Bilastine	Unlicensed	20 mg once daily
Cetirizine	1–2 years: 250 µg/kg twice daily (unlicensed) 2–6 years: 2.5 mg twice daily 6–12 years: 5 mg twice daily	10 mg once daily
Desloratadine	1–6 years: 1.25 mg once daily 6–12 years: 2.5 mg once daily	5 mg once daily
Fexofenadine	6–12 years: 30 mg bid (licensed for allergic rhinitis)	180 mg once daily
Loratadine	2–12 years, <30 kg: 5 mg once daily 2–12 years, >30 kg: 10 mg once daily	10 mg once daily
Mizolastine	Unlicensed	10 mg once daily
Rupatadine	Unlicensed	10 mg once daily (not available in UK)
Ebastine	2–5 years, 2.5 mg once daily 6–12 years, 5 mg once daily	10 mg once daily (not available in the UK)
Sedating antihistamines		
Alimemazine	6–24 months: 250 µg/kg (max 2.5 µg three to four times daily; specialist use only) (not licensed in UK for use in children under 2 years) 2–5 years: 2.5 mg three to four times daily 5–12 years: 5 mg three to four times daily	10 mg two to three times daily (max. 100 mg/day) *Elderly:* 10 mg once to twice daily
Chlorphenamine	1–24 months: 1 mg twice daily 2–6 years: 1 mg every 4–6 hours (max. 6 mg/day) 6–12 years: 2 mg every 4–6 hours (max. 12 mg/day)	4 mg every 4–6 hours (Max. 24 mg/day) *Elderly:* max. 12 mg/day
Diphenhydramine	2-6 years: every 4–6 hours (max. 5 mg/kg or 37.5 mg daily) 6–12 years: 12.5–25 mg every 4–6 hours (max. 150 mg daily)	25–50 mg every 4–6 hours (max. 300 mg/day) (not available in UK)
Hydroxyzine	6 month–6 years: 5–15 mg in divided doses (max. 2 mg/kg daily) 6–12 years 15–25 mg daily in divided doses increased to 2 mg/kg/day	25 mg at night (Up to 25 mg three to four times daily) *Elderly:* up to 25 mg twice daily
Promethazine	2–5 years: 5 mg twice daily (or 5–15 mg at night) 5–10 years: 5–10 mg mg twice daily (or 10–25 mg at night) >10 years: 10–20 mg twice daily (or 25 mg at night, up to 25 mg twice daily if required)	10–20 mg two to three times daily

ANTIHISTAMINES

Dermatologic prescribing

- See **Table 29.1** for dosage details.

Common problems

- Drowsiness may affect skilled tasks, e.g. driving, and patients should be cautioned regarding this risk

- First generation antihistamines may have substantial anticholinergic activity, requiring caution in those at risk for urinary retention, glaucoma, epilepsy, cardiac arrhythmias, hypotension, confusion, and dementia

- In patients with significantly impaired renal function, acrivastine, cetirizine, and levocetirizine should be avoided or used at reduced doses

- Mizolastine should be avoided in patients with prolonged QT intervals

SODIUM CROMOGLICATE

Dermatologic prescribing

- *<2 years:* 20 mg/kg/day divided into four doses

- *2–12 years:* 100 mg orally four times daily

- *Adults:* 200 mg four times daily before meals. If necessary, this may be increased after 2–3 weeks to a maximum dose of 40 mg/kg daily and then tapered as tolerated by the patient

Common problems

- Usually well tolerated. Not known to be harmful during pregnancy or lactation

LEUKOTRIENE RECEPTOR ANTAGONISTS (LTRA)

Dermatologic prescribing (montelukast)

- 2 months–5 years: 4 mg once daily in the evening

- 6–14 years: 5 mg once daily in the evening

- Adults and children >15 years: 10 mg once daily in the evening

Cautions

- There is limited evidence for the safe use of leukotriene receptor antagonists during pregnancy

- Be aware of drug interactions, e.g. zafirlukast increases the anticoagulant effect of warfarin

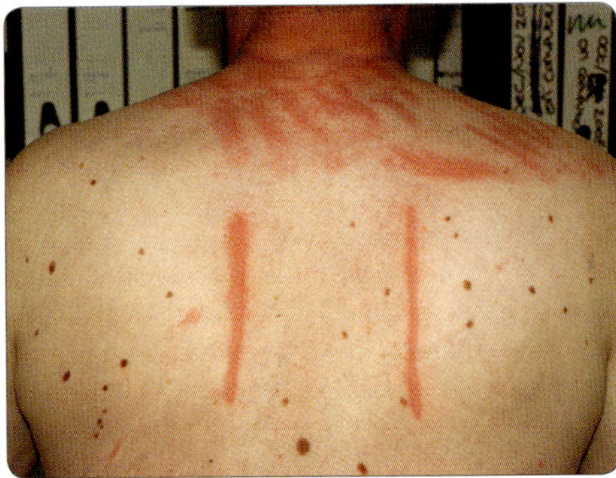

Figure 29.2 Dermatographic urticaria.

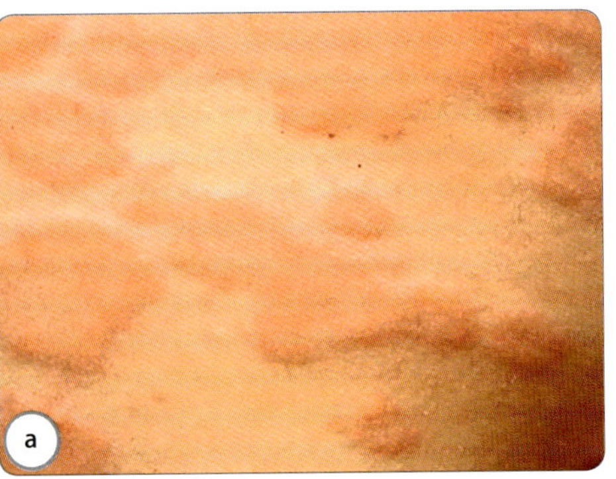

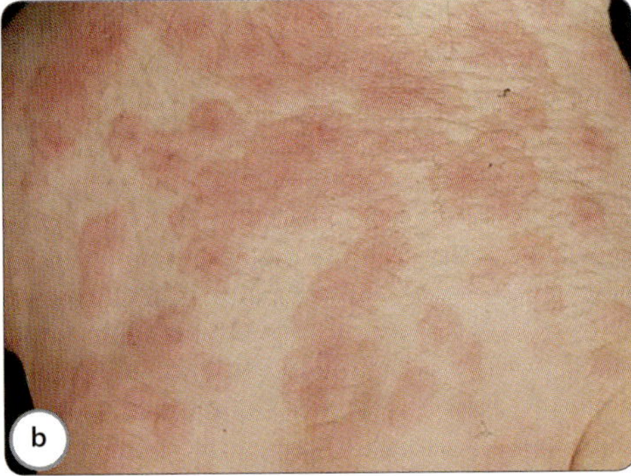

Figure 29.3 Urticaria versus erythema multiforme. Urticaria (a) is characterised by pruritic, annular, raised, erythematous wheals without scale. Note the pale centers. Erythema multiforme (b) is frequently mistaken for urticaria and vice versa. Note the raised pink plaques with dusky centers (target-like) and incipient central vesicle formation. Erythema multiforme is often tender and does not respond to antihistamines. Herpes and mycoplasma infections should be considered and if eruption is widespread, drug hypersensitivity reactions.

Common problems

- Side effects include gastrointestinal symptoms, elevated alanine aminotransferase (especially with zafirlukast), and neuropsychiatric problems, including nightmares and insomnia. Paraesthesia and arthralgia have also rarely been reported

Further reading

de Silva NL, Damayanthi H, Rajapakse AC, et al. Leukotriene receptor antagonists for chronic urticaria: a systematic review. Allergy Asthma Clin Immunol 2014; 10:24.

Leslie TA, Greaves MW, Yosipovitch G. Current topical and systemic therapies for itch. Handb Exp Pharmacol 2015; 226:337-56.

Leslie TA, Raap U. Urticaria. In: Misery L, Stander S (eds), Pruritus. London: Springer, 2016; pp 151-156.

Sharma M, Bennett C, Cohen SN, Carter B. H1-antihistamines for chronic spontaneous urticaria. Cochrane Database Syst Rev 2014; CD006137.

Zuberbier T, Aberer W, Asero R, et al. The EAACI/GA(2) LEN/EDF/WAO Guideline for the definition, classification, diagnosis, and management of urticaria: the 2013 revision and update. Allergy 2014; 69:868–887.

Mastocytosis treatment pearls

- Introducing sodium cromoglicate at slowly increasing doses may help reduce side effects such as headache, fatigue, nausea, diarrhea, arthralgia, and rash
- Sodium cromoglicate is more beneficial when used as an adjunct to other medications in systemic mastocytosis with bowel symptoms

Antimalarials

Dermatologic indications

- Cutaneous lupus erythematosus, dermatomyositis, porphyria cutanea tarda, polymorphic light eruption, granuloma annulare, sarcoidosis
- *Also used for:* solar urticaria, chronic erythema nodosum, lupus panniculitis, urticarial vasculitis, chronic graft-versus-host disease, lichen planus, oral lichen planus, reticular erythematous mucinosis, Jessner's lymphocytic infiltrate, pemphigus, atopic dermatitis

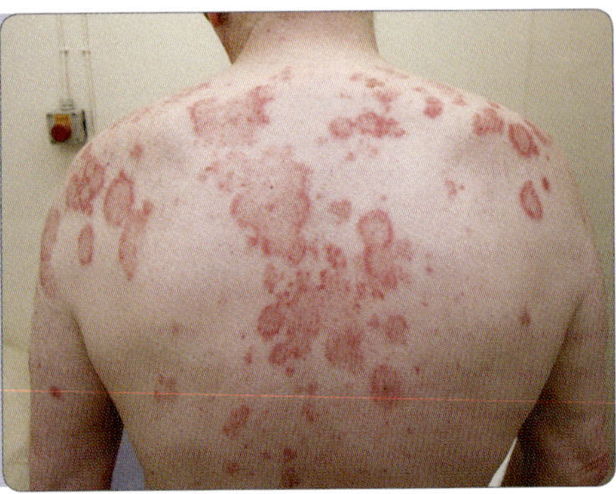

Figure 30.1 Subacute cutaneous lupus erythematosus with photosensitive, annular and polycyclic erythematous scaly plaques.

Background

Antimalarials have multiple mechanisms of action that are useful in treating dermatologic diseases:

- *Immunomodulatory:* inhibit autoantigen processing, leading to reduced stimulation of autoreactive CD4+ T-cells. Reduce macrophage production of IL-1, IL-2, IL-6, and TNF-α and T-cell production of IL-1, IL-2, and IL-5. Bind to DNA leading to competitive inhibition of anti-DNA antibodies
- *Anti-inflammatory:* inhibit phospholipase A2 and C as well as formation of IL-1-β and TNF-α. Inhibit mast cells and the Toll-like receptor 9 signal pathway
- *Antiproliferative:* interfere with protein synthesis
- *UV absorption:* inhibit UV-induced inflammatory reactions
- *Coagulation:* inhibit thrombocyte aggregation by diminishing CD41a and CD61 expression

Dermatologic prescribing

- *Route:* oral
- Dosing calculated by ideal body weight or real body weight up to a maximum dosage of 400 mg daily
  - Hydroxychloroquine: <6.5 mg/kg/day
  - Quinacrine (Mepacrine): compounded; 100 mg/day
  - Chloroquine: <3.5 mg/kg/day
- For hydroxychloroquine: if taller than 5 ft 2 in (158 cm), a patient typically needs 200 mg twice daily (may be given as a single daily dose if tolerated). If a patient is shorter than 5 ft 2 in (158 cm), they will often need 200–300 mg daily
- For most patients, hydroxychloroquine should be started at the maximum dose allowed by weight, and the response then evaluated after 3 months. If no improvements are seen after 3 months, quinacrine can be added, or chloroquine substituted
- The typical dose of chloroquine is 250 mg/day
- For porphyria cutanea tarda, much lower doses of hydroxychloroquine and chloroquine are used: hydroxychloroquine 100 mg twice weekly or chloroquine 125 mg twice weekly

Cautions

- *Retinopathy:* those with known retinopathy should avoid hydroxychloroquine and chloroquine, as they can cause retinopathy, in some cases after years of use. Chloroquine has a higher risk of ocular toxicity than hydroxychloroquine
- *Medication interaction:* antimalarials have multiple drug interactions; potential interactions should be assessed in all patients. Ampicillin, cyclosporine, digoxin, and ranitidine are common drugs that interact with antimalarials
- *Pregnancy/lactation risk:* antimalarials cross the placenta and reach the fetus. Several studies have assessed the safety of these drugs during pregnancy, and none have detected a greater risk of congenital malformations or ocular, neurologic, or auditory toxicity. The benefit of controlling the underlying disease and avoiding flares must be weighed against the potential risks of medication use

Common problems

- Gastrointestinal upset, diarrhea, headache, and insomnia or altered dreams
- Ocular toxicity (associated with higher doses):

- *Reversible:* corneal deposition, loss of accommodation, retinal pigment deposition
- *Irreversible:* retinopathy (chloroquine > hydroxychloroquine; not seen with quinacrine)

■ Cutaneous adverse reactions: blue-gray pigmentation (10–30% with hydroxychloroquine and chloroquine), morbilliform, lichenoid or urticarial eruptions, exfoliative reactions, DRESS syndrome, and hair lightening and thinning. Quinacrine frequently causes yellowish discoloration of the skin and sclera

Further reading

Kalia S, Dutz JP. New concepts in antimalarial use and mode of action in dermatology. Dermatol Ther 2007; 20:160–174.

Kuhn A, Ruland V, Bonsmann G. Cutaneous lupus erythematosus: update of therapeutic options part I. J Am Acad Dermatol 2011; 65:e179–193.

Rodriguez-Caruncho C, Bielsa Marsol I. Antimalarials in dermatology: mechanism of action, indications, and side effects. Actas Dermosifiliogr 2014; 105:243–252.

Treatment pearls

■ Screening for retinopathy:
- Very low risk, increases with cumulative dose: <1–7/1000 users, 1–5% after 5–7 years, higher after 15–20 years
- In many countries, baseline screening with ophthalmology is mandatory when initiating treatment with hydroxychloroquine or chloroqine. In other countries, visual acuity testing alone is performed in the dermatology clinic prior to initiation
- Recommendations for the frequency of follow-up screening vary. Some guidelines suggest that annual screening may commence 5 years after initiation of therapy. In many centers, however, annual screening is recommended while on hydroxychloroquine and twice yearly screening while on chloroquine starting upon therapy initiation.

■ Laboratory monitoring: a complete blood count and liver and renal function should be assessed at baseline and every 6–12 months thereafter

■ Antimalarials typically take 3 months before their effect is clinically apparent

■ Although chloroquine is considered to be more efficacious than hydroxychloroquine, it has a higher risk of retinal toxicity

■ Quinacrine (mepacrine) can be added to hydroxychloroquine or chloroquine as it has no increased risk of retinal toxicity. Hydroxychloroquine and chloroquine should not be combined given additive ocular toxicity. Quinacrine has a risk of aplastic anemia, which may be preceded by lichen planus-like eruption. In addition, quinacrine has a rare risk of transaminitis. A complete blood count and hepatic function should be performed 2–4 weeks after initiation of quinacrine

■ Smoking has been associated with decreased efficacy of antimalarials in some studies. Smoking cessation should be encouraged

■ Patients with dermatomyositis are more likely to develop a cutaneous drug eruption to hydroxychloroquine, most often a morbilliform eruption, with rates as high as 30%

■ Antimalarials can rarely affect the muscles, including the heart, causing a myopathy; if suspected, electron microscopy can confirm the diagnosis

Dermatologic indications

- Oral ivermectin is an antihelminthic agent approved to treat intestinal strongyloidiasis (*Strongyloides stercoralis*), onchocerciasis (*Onchocerca volvulus*), and pediculosis capitis (head lice). It is also used to treat scabies and cutaneous larva migrans

- Ivermectin 1% topical cream is used to treat inflammatory rosacea

- Ivermectin 0.5% lotion is used to treat pediculosis capitis

- Albendazole is an antihelminthic and antiprotozoal agent used to treat neurocysticercosis and hydatid disease (echinococcosis). It is also used to treat infections caused by *Ascaris lumbricoides*, *Enterobius vermicularis* (pinworm), *Ancylostoma duodenale*, *Trichuris trichiura* (whipworm), and *Necator americanus* (hookworm). Occasionally, it can be used for *Giardia* infections

- Mebendazole is primarily used to treat gastrointestinal (GI) nematode infections, such as pinworm and hookworm infections, and the intestinal form of toxocariasis (prior to its spread into tissues beyond the GI tract). It is no longer available in the US

Background

Ivermectin selectively interacts with glutamate-gated chloride channels on the muscles and nerves of parasites. This causes increased permeability of cell membranes, leading to paralysis and death of the parasite.

Albendazole and mebendazole selectively bind beta-tubulin polymerase, disrupting microtubule formation with subsequent paralysis and death of the parasite.

Dermatologic prescribing

Ivermectin

- *Oral:* 3 mg tablets with weight-based dosing. When oral ivermectin is prescribed off-label for scabies, the US Centers for Disease Control and Prevention recommends a single dose of 200 µg/kg, repeated after 2 weeks. Doses typically range from 3–15 mg depending on the patient's weight. Crusted scabies usually requires additional doses. Occasionally, doses of 250–400 µg/kg may be needed. The dose for treating pediculosis is 400 µg/kg given on day 1 and day 8. Patients should be advised to take the tablets on an empty stomach with water

- *Topical:* 1% cream. A thin film should be applied to the affected areas of the face once daily for inflammatory rosacea

Albendazole

- *Oral:* 200 mg tablets; patients should be advised to take with food

Mebendazole

- Pinworms (threadworms): Adults and children >2 years treated with 100 mg as a single dose, repeated after 2 weeks for reinfections

- Whipworms: Adults and children >2 years treated with 100 mg twice daily for 3 days

Cautions

Ivermectin

- A Mazzotti-like reaction can rarely occur (fever, pruritus, urticarial rash, arthralgia, synovitis, lymph node enlargement or tenderness)

- An ophthalmic reaction can rarely occur (conjunctivitis, limbitis, eyelid edema, or vision changes)

- Caution should be observed in patients with a history of seizures. p-Glycoprotein restricts ivermectin from crossing the blood-brain barrier. Deficiency of p-glycoprotein may cause a risk of neurotoxicity (ataxia, seizures)

- Patients taking the oral form should be instructed to rise slowly from a sitting/supine position as the drug may cause orthostatic hypotension

- Ivermectin may enhance anticoagulation when combined with vitamin K antagonists including warfarin

- Use should be avoided during pregnancy and lactation and in children weighing <15 kg

Albendazole

- Rare and serious adverse effects include bone marrow suppression, aplastic anemia, agranulocytosis, angioedema, and Stevens–Johnson syndrome

- Carbamazepine, phenytoin, and phenobarbital decrease the half-life and lower the plasma concentration of albendazole. Cimetidine, praziquantel, and dexamethasone increase the half-life and raise the plasma concentration of albendazole. Albendazole inhibits theophylline metabolism, and levels should be monitored

- Caution should be observed in patients with hepatic or biliary disease
- Use should be avoided during pregnancy and in children less than 1 year old

Mebendazole

- Allergic-type reactions may occur including urticarial rash, angioedema, pruritus, and flushing
- Elevated serum transaminases and rare cases of acute liver injury have been associated with high dose therapy

Common problems

- Common side effects of all three agents are gastrointestinal (nausea, vomiting, diarrhea), neurologic (dizziness, headache), and hematologic (leukopenia)

Further reading

Chosidow O. Clinical practices. Scabies. N Engl J Med 2006; 354:1718–1727.

Chouela EN, Abeldaño AM, Pellerano G, et al. Equivalent therapeutic efficacy and safety of ivermectin and lindane in the treatment of human scabies. Arch Dermatol 1999; 135:651–655.

Dourmishev AL, Dourmishev LA, Schwartz RA. Ivermectin: pharmacology and application in dermatology. Int J Dermatol 2005; 44:981–988.

Treatment pearls

Ivermectin

- Ivermectin can be combined with topical scabicides and keratolytics for the treatment of crusted scabies
- Randomized trials and clinical experience suggest that ivermectin is safe and may be considered in patients with scabies who fail topical therapy or have difficulty complying with treatment
- Follow up clinical evaluations with scrapings and stool examinations are recommended, depending on the organism being treated

Albendazole

- A pregnancy test should be performed prior to initiation of therapy. Pregnancy is contraindicated until 1 month following completion of therapy. Contraception should be discussed with all patients starting albendazole
- A complete blood count and hepatic panel should be undertaken before starting treatment and every 2 weeks thereafter while on therapy

Mebendazole

- Pinworm (threadworm) should be considered in any patient with nocturnal pruritus ani or vulvae, particularly in a child

Antiviral agents

Dermatologic indications

- *Acyclovir, famciclovir, valacyclovir:* primary or recurrent herpes simplex (HSV) infections of skin or mucous membranes; prophylaxis for recurrent HSV infection, herpes encephalitis, neonatal herpes; varicella zoster virus (VZV) infections. Famciclovir is licenced for genital herpes and herpes zoster

- *Ganciclovir:* prevention of cytomegalovirus (CMV) reactivation following transplant, life-threatening or sight-threatening CMV infection in immunocompromised patients

- *Widely used for:* eczema herpeticum, recurrent erythema multiforme, varicella (chickenpox), zoster (shingles) (acyclovir, famciclovir, valacyclovir) and reactivation of other herpes infections, e.g. CMV, EBV, HHV-6, and HHV-7 in immunosuppressed patients (ganciclovir)

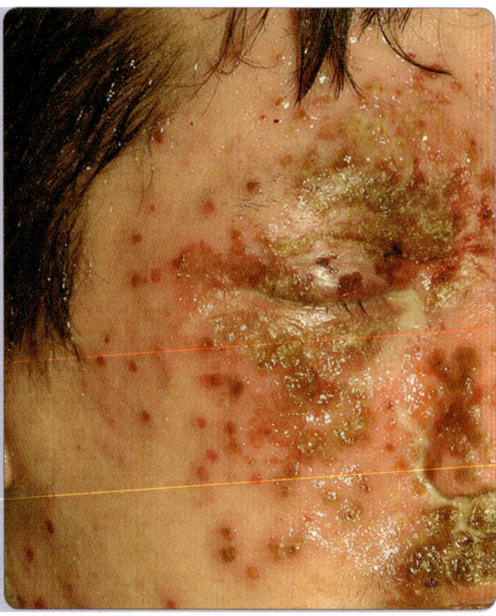

Figure 32.1 Eczema herpeticum (Kaposi's varcelliform eruption). HSV spread diffusely on the face of an individual with atopic dermatitis. Note the monomorphic erosions with crusting of older herpes blisters (around orbit and upper lip) and vesiculation (laterally). Secondary infection with *Staphylococcus aureus* is often also found.

Background

These drugs are activated by viral thymidine kinases (TKs) (for mechanisms see **Chapter 7**). Rarely, mutation of a viral TK gene may lead to resistance. The viral TKs of VZV and CMV are less efficient at converting the drugs to the monophosphate forms than the TK of herpes simplex, making these drugs less effective in these infections.

Valacyclovir is a prodrug of acyclovir; famciclovir is a prodrug of penciclovir. Conversion to the active form occurs rapidly in the human cell. The prodrug of ganciclovir, valganciclovir, is also available.

Primary HSV infections are often subclinical but may present with local pain, blistering, and erosions, often with systemic symptoms. Recurrent episodes are less severe than clinically evident primary infection, and occur as often as monthly or as infrequently as once in a lifetime. Triggers include local trauma, sunlight, other infections, and immunosuppression.

Primary VZV infection causes generalized chickenpox, whereas recurrence of VZV infection presents as zoster. Recurrence is more likely with older age or immunosuppression.

Primary CMV infection is usually subclinical, but may rarely present with an infectious mononucleosis-like disease. Reactivation of CMV in immunosuppression can be detected by PCR of blood and may present with systemic symptoms and occasionally purpura, skin nodules, or ulceration. Drug reaction with eosinophilia and systemic symptoms (DRESS) may be associated with CMV, EBV, HHV-6, or HHV-7 reactivation.

Dermatologic prescribing

- Acyclovir, famciclovir and valacyclovir can be administered orally; acyclovir and ganciclovir intravenously

- Shorter, higher-dose regimens may be as effective as longer, lower-dose regimens, but full comparison studies have not been conducted

Primary HSV gingivostomatitis or genitalis

- Oral acyclovir (200 mg 5 times daily, 400 mg 3 times daily, or 800 mg twice daily), famciclovir (250 mg 3 times daily) or valacyclovir (500–1000 mg twice daily) for 7–10 days

Recurrent HSV labialis or genitalis

- Oral acyclovir (200 mg 5 times daily or 400–800 mg 3 times daily for 5 days), famciclovir (125 mg or 500 mg 2× daily for 5 days or single 1500 mg dose) or valacyclovir (500 mg 2× daily for 3 days or 2000 mg 2× daily for 1 day)

Recurrent HSV labialis or genitalis in immunocompromised patients

- Oral acyclovir (400 mg 4× daily) or IV (5 mg/kg every 8 hours), oral famciclovir (500 mg twice daily) or valacyclovir 1000 mg 2× daily for 5–7 days

Prophylaxis for frequent/severe recurrent disease

- Oral acyclovir (400 mg 2× daily), famciclovir (125 mg 3× times daily or 250 mg 2× daily) or valacyclovir (250 mg 2× daily or 500 mg once daily) for 6–12 months

- If immunosuppressed, the dose should be increased (e.g. acyclovir 400 mg 4× daily, famciclovir 500 mg 2× daily, valacyclovir 500 mg twice daily)

Neonatal HSV

- IV acyclovir (60 mg/kg/day in 3 divided doses for 2–3 weeks) followed by oral acyclovir for 6 months

Chickenpox (varicella zoster virus)

- Antiviral treatment is not usually necessary in children, but in adults consider oral acyclovir (20 mg/kg/day, up to a total dose of 800 mg 5× daily) or valacyclovir (1000 mg 3× daily) for 7 days
- Chickenpox in immunosuppressed or suspected encephalitis: acyclovir 5–10 mg/kg or 500 mg/m^2 8-hourly, IV for 2–10 days followed by oral dosing

Zoster (shingles)

- Oral acyclovir (800 mg 5× daily), famciclovir (250–500 mg 3× daily) or 750 mg 2× daily, or valacyclovir (1000 mg 3× daily) for 7–10 days
- Zoster in immunosuppressed patients: oral acyclovir (800 mg 5× daily or IV 10 mg/kg 8-hourly, IV for 2–10 days followed by oral dosing for a total of 7–10 days). Alternatively, famciclovir 500 mg 3× daily or valacyclovir 1000 mg 3× daily for 10 days

CMV in immunocompromised patients

- Ganciclovir IV (5 mg/kg 2× daily for 7–14 days)

Cautions

- In renal impairment, the dose of oral or infused antiviral should be reduced, calculated according to creatinine clearance. As a broad rule, if the GFR is < 10 mL/min, a 5× daily dosing is reduced to 3× per day, a 3× daily dosing is reduced to 2× daily and a 2× daily dosing is reduced to once daily. In moderate renal impairment, the dose reduction may be intermediate
- The drugs are not licenced for use in pregnancy, but may be used if benefit outweighs risk. Antivirals are excreted in breast milk; babies of

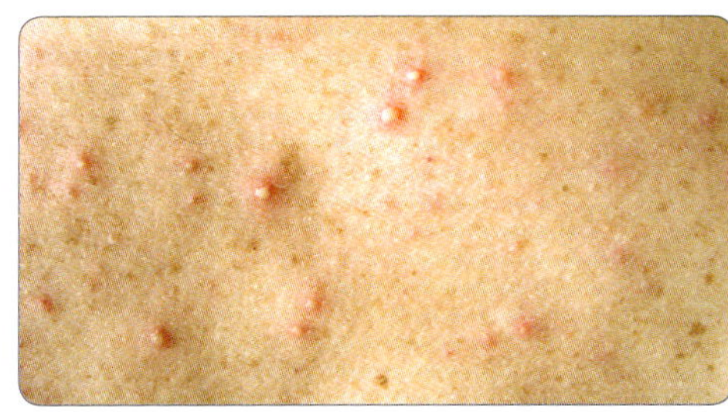

Figure 32.2 2–4 mm vesicles beginning to pustulate in chickenpox in an immunocompromised adult.

breastfeeding mothers will receive a low dose, estimated as 2% of the mother's dose. Acyclovir has no proven associations with fetal harm

- Adverse reactions to acyclovir, famciclovir, valacyclovir, or ganciclovir are rare; however, as the drugs are closely related, a reaction to one may induce cross reaction to another

Common problems

- Acyclovir, famciclovir and valacyclovir are usually well tolerated. The most common side effects are nausea, vomiting, diarrhea, headache. Rarely, vertigo, confusion, edema, arthralgia, rash, pruritus, or renal impairment may occur. With high doses or prolonged use, bone marrow suppression may be seen
- Ganciclovir can also cause myelosuppression, shortness of breath, and transient liver enzyme elevation
- Ganciclovir may interact with: didanosine, imipenem, mycophenolate mofetil, probenecid and zidovudine

Further reading

Cernik C, Gallina K, Brodell RT. The treatment of herpes simplex infections: an evidence-based review. Arch Intern Med 2008; 168:1137–1144.

Johnston C, Saracino M, Kuntz S, et al. Standard-dose and high-dose daily antiviral therapy for short episodes of genital HSV-2 reactivation: three randomized, open-label, cross-over trials. Lancet 2012; 379:641–647.

Treatment pearls

- Anti-viral medications should be started as early as possible in the disease course
- When skin lesions are active viral shedding is high, and isolation measures to avoid infection of immunocompromised (including pregnant) individuals should be taken
- Eczema herpeticum can be treated as per the regimens above for zoster
- Erythema multiforme with a known or suspected HSV trigger is treatable with antiviral prophylaxis

Azathioprine

Dermatologic indications

- Immunobullous diseases (e.g. pemphigus vulgaris, bullous pemphigoid)
- Cutaneous small vessel vasculitis, cutaneous polyarteritis nodosa
- Atopic dermatitis (atopic eczema)
- Cutaneous lupus erythematosus, cutaneous dermatomyositis
- Chronic actinic dermatitis
- *Also used for:* psoriasis, pyoderma gangrenosum, chronic urticaria

Background

Azathioprine inhibits purine synthesis after conversion to the active metabolite 6-thioguanine monophosphate and other salts.

It suppresses T-cell mediated function and reduces antibody production by B-cells.

Dermatologic prescribing

- For patients with normal levels of thiopurine methyltransferase (TMPT), azathioprine is typically given at a dose of 1–2.5 mg/kg/day
- *Route:* oral
- *Dosage forms:* azathioprine is available in 50 mg, 75 mg, and 100 mg tablets
- *Monitoring:* when TPMT testing is normal, a complete blood count with differential and liver function tests may be completed at 2 weeks and 6 weeks after initiation of therapy and then every 8 weeks thereafter. In the absence of TMPT testing, measurement of a complete blood count with differential and liver function should occur weekly for 4 weeks after initiation of therapy and then every month

Cautions

Hematologic

- Cytopenias, particularly in patients with low TMPT (most often lymphopenia and leukopenia)

Malignancy

- Post-transplantation lymphoproliferative disease or lymphoma
- Hepatosplenic T-cell lymphoma in patients with inflammatory bowel disease, particularly those also treated with tumor necrosis factor-alpha (TNF-α) antagonists
- Non-melanoma skin cancer, particularly squamous cell carcinoma

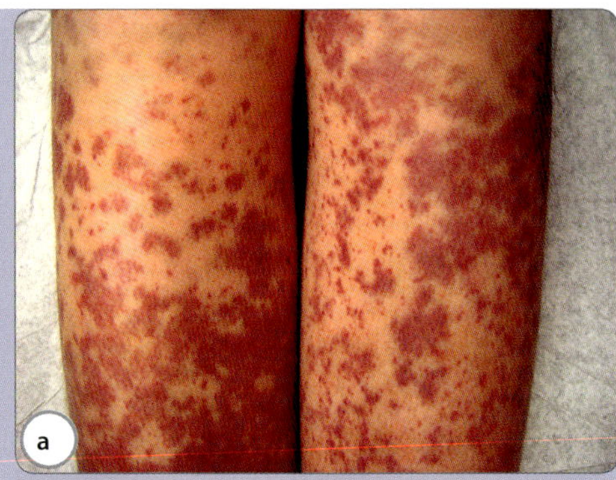

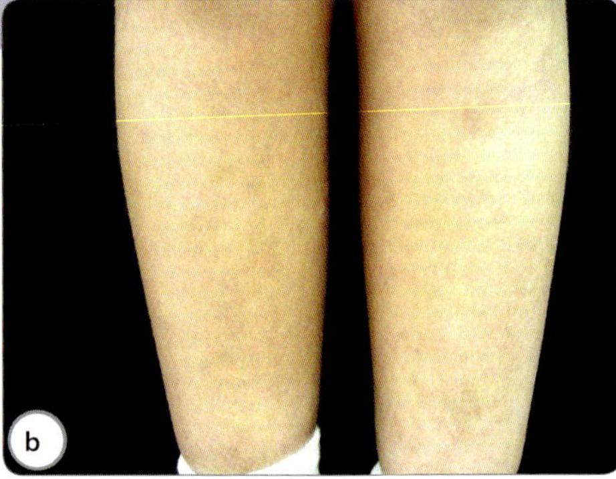

Figure 33.1 Leukocytoclastic vasculitis (a) before and (b) after azathioprine.

Idiosyncratic reactions

- Hypersensitivity reaction characterized by fever, hepatitis, vascular collapse, generalized rash
- Induction of acute febrile neutrophilic dermatosis (Sweet's syndrome)

Medication interactions

- Allopurinol and febuxostat are xanthine oxidase inhibitors and increase the risk of cytopenias and possibly the level of immune suppression when given concomitantly with azathioprine; these are therefore typically avoided in patients taking azathioprine
- Angiotensin converting enzyme inhibitors increase the risk of leukopenia
- Mesalamine (mesalazine) blocks the degradation of active metabolites, thereby increasing the immunosuppressive effects
- Azathioprine may decrease the anticoagulant effect of warfarin

Pregnancy/lactation risk

- Although azathioprine has been considered to have evidence of risk in pregnancy, it is often not stopped during pregnancy in patients with organ transplantation. In addition, it is frequently used in patients with systemic lupus erythematosus during pregnancy. Risks should be carefully weighed up against the benefits

- The risk in lactation is unknown, but most sources recommend alternative therapy if possible

Immunosuppression

- Concomitant use of other immunosuppressive therapy with azathioprine increases the risk of infection and level of immune suppression

Common problems

- Nausea and vomiting are common complications

- Anorexia may occur in some patients

- Transaminitis (elevated AST and/or ALT) occurs in some patients, but when less than 2–3 fold (the upper limits of normal) does not warrant alteration of the dose or cessation of therapy

- Acute pancreatitis is a rare but important adverse event

Further reading

Badalamenti SS, Kerdel FA. Azathioprine. In: Wolverton SE (Ed). Comprehensive Dermatologic Therapy, 3rd Edn. Philadelphia: Elsevier-Saunders, 2012:182–189.

Roekevisch E, Spuls PI, Kuester D, et al. Efficacy and safety of systemic treatments for moderate-to-severe atopic dermatitis: a systematic review. J Allergy Clin Immunol 2014; 133:429–438.

Thomsen SF, Karlsmark T, Clemmensen KK, et al. Outcome of treatment with azathioprine in severe atopic dermatitis: a 5-year retrospective study of adult outpatients. Br J Dermatol 2015; 172:1122–1124.

Zhao CY, Murrell DF. Pemphigus vulgaris: an evidence-based treatment update. Drugs 2015; 75:271–284.

Treatment pearls

- It is ideal to test thiopurine methyltransferase (TPMT) prior to prescribing. Patients with very low levels of TPMT (homozygotes) should not be given azathioprine, those with medium levels (heterozygotes) should be dosed at lower levels (1 mg/kg/day), and those with normal levels are dosed at 2–2.5 mg/kg/day. There are some patients with very high levels that may benefit from higher doses of azathioprine

- Normal TPMT activity does not preclude life threatening myelotoxicity, so monitoring blood counts routinely is still critical

- In patients with suspected hypersensitivity reactions, do not re-administer azathioprine or 6-mercaptopurine, as there is a high likelihood of cardiovascular collapse

- The onset of action for azathioprine in dermatologic disease is roughly 12 weeks at 'full' dose. Cessation prior to that time is an inadequate trial

- Although non-melanoma skin cancer is linked to azathioprine use in allograft recipients, its linkage in patients with dermatologic disease is not as well established. Recent studies of patients with inflammatory bowel disease treated with azathioprine have demonstrated an increased likelihood of cutaneous malignancy, but this potential association may be heightened by concomitant or subsequent use of TNF antagonists

- Following control of disease, gradual reduction and possible cessation of therapy is possible, but should be done slowly

- For patients with pemphigus, monitoring levels of antibodies to desmogleins may indicate when it is safe to reduce dosage levels

- Recent evidence suggests that careful combination with allopurinol may allow a lower dose of azathioprine to be used, with the aim of reducing the potentially adverse long term effects of azathioprine. However, this is rarely done in clinical practice

Dermatologic indications

- Plaque psoriasis
- Moderate to severe psoriasis requiring systemic therapy, usually when standard systemic therapy (e.g. methotrexate) has failed or cannot be used; in many centers, biologics are now being used first-line for moderate to severe psoriasis
- Refractory, localized disease occurring at high impact sites (face, hands, genital area, nails)
- *Also used for:* psoriasis variants (e.g. pustular psoriasis, erythrodermic psoriasis), pityriasis rubra pilaris, hidradenitis suppurativa, pyoderma gangrenosum, Behçet's disease, Netherton syndrome

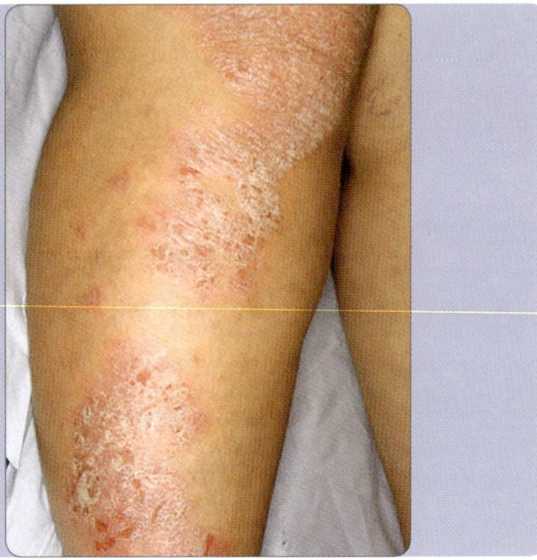

Figure 34.1 Biologic therapies have transformed the outcomes of patients with severe psoriasis.

Background

Short-term data (up to 1 year) indicate marked efficacy (**Table 34.1**) and tolerability and an excellent safety profile.

Infection, particularly reactivation of latent tuberculosis, may complicate therapy.

Additional long-term data is required to fully elucidate the overall safety profile, particularly in relation to malignancy risk.

Challenges include:

- Immunogenicity and the development of anti-drug antibodies, leading to gradual loss of efficacy
- Administration (subcutaneous injection for most agents or intravenous infusion for infliximab)
- High cost

Targets for currently licensed biologics:

- Tumor necrosis factor (TNF): infliximab, adalimumab, etanercept
- p40 shared subunit of interleukin (IL) 12/23: ustekinumab
- IL-17: secukinumab, brodalumab
- IL-17A: ixekizumab

Biosimilar antibodies have the same basic amino-acid structure and target the same pathogenic molecule, but may have subtle differences in secondary and tertiary structures, therefore requiring robust pharmacovigilance. Debate is ongoing regarding the licensing of these products; currently, these products need to undergo the same level of clinical trial investigation pre-license. The availability of biosimilar TNF-antagonists should reduce cost and therefore improve treatment access.

Dermatologic prescribing

- Dosing is usually according to license (**Table 34.1**)

Use of anti-TNF therapy in other skin diseases:

- Recent clinical trial data has supported the role of anti-TNF therapy in hidradenitis suppurativa (HS) at disease specific doses (e.g. adalimumab is now licensed at 160 mg week 0, then 80 mg at week 2, then 40 mg at week 4 followed by 40 mg weekly).
- Anti-TNF therapy is also useful in pyoderma gangrenosum (especially inflammatory bowel disease associated), Behçet's disease, pityriasis rubra pilaris and Netherton syndrome

Cautions

- *People at higher risk of infection:* elderly, those with multiple co-morbidities (e.g diabetes, chronic lung disease), on co-therapy with other immunosuppressive agents, or on higher doses of biologic therapy. Patients with HIV, hepatitis and bone marrow disorders
- *Patients at risk of tuberculosis:* It is imperative to screen for latent mycobacterium tuberculosis prior to commencement of therapy. Reactivation of tuberculosis or development of a serious infection should prompt immediate cessation of biologic therapy treatment
- *Active or previous malignancy:* biologic therapy is contraindicated unless the malignancy is low risk and/or adequately treated. In general,

Table 34.1 Overview and dosing schedule

Drug name	Drug type	Dosing schedule*	Efficacy (% clear or nearly clear)*‡
Infliximab	Chimeric human–murine monoclonal anti-TNF antibody	5 mg/kg intravenous infusion at week 0, 2, 6, and then every 8 weeks	82% (week 10)
Etanercept	Fusion protein composed of an extracellular ligand binding portion of the TNF receptor fused to the Fc portion of human IgG1	50 mg subcutaneous injection once weekly	32–39% (week 12)
Adalimumab	Fully human IgG1 anti-TNF antibody	40 mg subcutaneous injection week 0, 1, and then every 2 weeks	62.2% (week 16)
Ustekinumab	Fully human IgG1 κ monoclonal antibody which binds to the shared p40 protein subunit of the cytokines IL-12 and 23	Weight ≤100 kg (220 lb): 45 mg week 0, 4 ,12, and then every 3 months Weight >100 kg (220 lb): 90 mg week 0, 4 , 12, and then every 12 weeks	67.5% (week 16)
Secukinumab	Fully human IgG1 antibody which selectively binds and neutralizes IL-17A	100 mg week 0, 1, 2, 3, 4, and then every 4 weeks	82.9% (week 16)
Ixekizumab	Humanized IL-17A antagonist	160 mg at week 0, then 80 mg at weeks 2, 4, 6, 8, 10, and 12, and then 80 mg every 4 weeks	81–83% (week 12)

*See summary of product characteristics (SPC) for regulatory prescribing information

‡Trials not directly comparable. Data refers to those patients achieving physicians global assessment (PGA) 0-1

non-melanoma skin cancers and malignancies treated more than 5 years previously are not a contraindication to biologic therapy

- *Pregnancy/lactation:* biologic therapies are actively transported across the placenta during the second and third trimester (with measurable drug levels in infants) and are also secreted in breast milk. Their use should be avoided when possible, unless benefits to the mother clearly outweigh potential and currently uncertain risks (for example, impact on fetal and neonatal development and risk of infection)

- *Vaccination:* live attenuated virus vaccines must be avoided while on biologic therapy due to the risk of uninhibited viral/bacterial replication

Cautions

- *Moderate/severe cardiac failure:* (New York Grade III/IV) as TNF is implicated in the pathogenesis of cardiac failure in animal models

- *Demyelinating disorders:* Personal history or first-degree relative with demyelinating disorders due to a possible causal association

with TNF-antagonists and the development of demyelinating disease

Adverse effects

Common

- *Injection site reactions:* transient edema, pain, erythema

- *Infusion reactions (infliximab):* urticaria, angioedema, anaphylaxis

- *Infections:* upper respiratory tract, skin and soft tissue

- *Loss of long-term efficacy over time.* This can be due to the development of anti-drug antibodies (ADAs)

Uncommon

- *Adverse skin reactions:* paradoxical palmoplantar pustulosis or psoriasiform eruption, severe exfoliative dermatitis

- *Candida:* an increased rate of mucocutaneous candida infections are seen with anti-IL-17 therapy

Table 34.2 Suggested assessments at baseline and follow-up visits

Baseline assessment	Assessment every 3–6 months	Annual assessment
History to include risk assessment for infection, history of previous malignancy, congestive heart failure, demyelinating disorders	History to include assessment of infections, night sweats, unintentional weight loss, or any new symptoms	History to include assessment of infections, night sweats, unintentional weight loss, or any new symptoms

Physical examination:
    Lymphadenopathy
    Hepatosplenomegaly
    Full skin exam
	Repeat as clinically indicated	Full skin examination

Assessment and relevant screening investigations for latent tuberculosis:
    Chest X-ray
    Mantoux test (PPD)/IFN-γ release assay
	Repeat as clinically indicated	Mantoux test (PPD)/IFN-γ release assay

Full blood count Renal function Liver function	Full blood count Renal function Liver function	Full blood count Renal function Liver function
HIV Hepatitis B, Hepatitis C ANA Varicella (VZV) †		Consider repeat testing in people who belong to groups at increased risk of infection

Vaccinations:
    Pneumococcal
    Influenza
 	
In certain individuals:
    Hepatitis B vaccination§
    VZV vaccination if non-immune§
		Advise annual influenza vaccination
		Reminder to avoid live vaccines

Ensure patient is enrolled in relevant cancer screening programs based on local guidelines		Ensure patient is enrolled in relevant cancer screening programs based on local guidelines

* According to local policy; † if no definite history of prior VZV infection; § if seronegative

- *TNF tumor necrosis factor (TNF)-α antagonist-induced lupus-like syndrome (TAILS):* has been reported, more commonly with etanercept and infliximab. Features include cutaneous lesions (malar rash, discoid rash, photosensitivity), arthritis, serositis, oral ulcers, hematologic abnormalities, and positive autoantibodies. Notably, TNF-antagonists may induce auto-antibodies in many patients, but only rarely are these of clinical significance

Uncertain risk

Malignancy: long-term safety registries should help further define potential lifetime risk.

Further reading

National Institute for Health and Care Excellence. NICE guidelines CG 153. Psoriasis: Assessment and Management. London: NICE, 2012.

Smith CH, Anstey AV, Barker JN, et al. British Association of Dermatologists' guidelines for biologic interventions for psoriasis 2009. Br J Dermatol 2009; 161:987–1019.

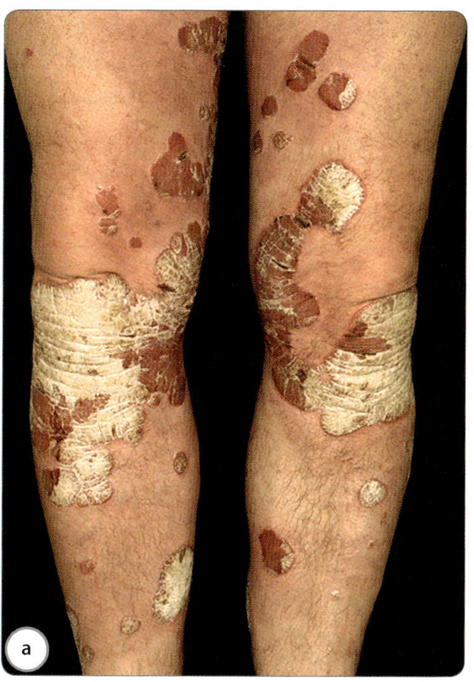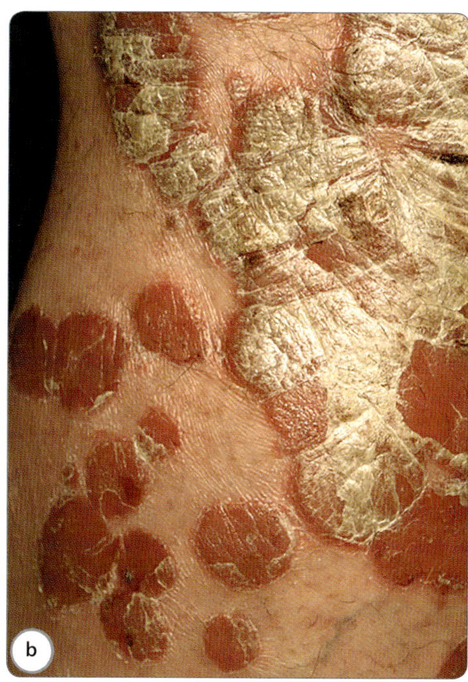

Figure 34.2 (a) Chronic plaque psoriasis of the legs showing thick micaceous scale. (b) Close up of psoriatic plaque showing clear demarcation of plaque border and adherent scale.

Treatment pearls

- In patients with psoriatic arthritis, assess disease activity in both skin and joints. Skin and joints may respond independently
- Risk of demyelination appears to be specific to TNF-antagonists
- Ustekinumab or secukinumab may be used in patients with a history of or active demyelinating disease
- Patients with primary failure of, or lack of response to one class of drug (for example TNF antagonists), may respond better to biologic therapy that targets an alternative pathway (IL12/23, IL17)
- Methotrexate combined with biologic therapy may reduce the production of anti-drug antibodies in addition to maximizing therapeutic response. Consider this approach in patients with rapid secondary failure to biologic therapy
- Transaminitis may be seen with biologic therapy. Rarely, autoimmune hepatitis may occur
- Biologic therapy may reduce vaccine immunogenicity (influenza, pneumococcal), however, the response is still sufficient enough to warrant vaccination
- The clinical presentation of infection in patients on biologic therapy may be atypical, warranting a high index of suspicion. Extra-pulmonary manifestations of tuberculosis are more common with TNF-antagonists
- Patients receiving biologic therapy should ideally be registered in a pharmacovigilance registry in order to assess the long-term safety of these treatments

MONOCLONAL ANTIBODIES

Dermatologic indications

- Ipilimumab, pembrolizumab and nivolumab are EMA, MHRA, and FDA approved for metastatic and unresectable, locally advanced melanoma

Background

Ipilimumab binds and deactivates CTLA-4 (inhibitor of T-cell activation), thereby upregulating T-cell immune responses nonspecifically.

Pembrolizumab and nivolumab block PD-1 (negative regulator of T-cell function) and thereby allow T-cells to become more easily activated to kill tumor cells.

Dermatologic prescribing

- Ipilimumab: 3 mg/kg every 4 weeks as an infusion for a total of four doses
- Pembrolizumab: 2 mg/kg every 3 weeks
- Nivolumab: 3 mg/kg every 2 weeks

Cautions

- *Renal:* no dosage adjustment is needed for baseline renal impairment
- *Hepatic:* there are no guidelines for dosage adjustment for baseline hepatotoxicity, but given that hepatotoxicity is a known side effect and that worsening transaminitis will change the treatment course, caution is warranted
- *Pregnancy/lactation:* both are contraindicated

Common problems

- Almost all common side effects are secondary to the profound induced immune response
- A diffuse, maculopapular rash is often the first observed side effect, occurring after 3–4 weeks of therapy with a spectrum of severity. Topical corticosteroids and oral antihistamines can provide relief from the associated pruritus
- Vitiligo occurs in some patients, which is thought to possibly represent the appropriately heightened immune response to melanocytes, signaling a favorable response
- Severe hypersensitivity reactions, such as Stevens–Johnson syndrome or toxic epidermal necrolysis, are also rarely observed
- Colitis and diarrhea are seen commonly in a spectrum of severity with substantial effects on quality of life. Hepatotoxicity is also observed,

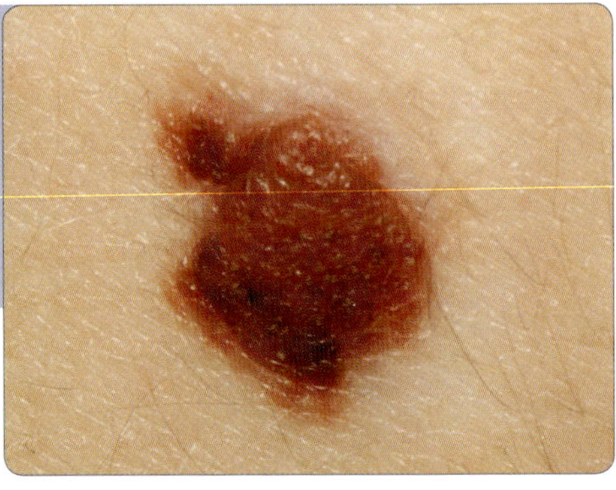

Figure 35.1 Malignant melanoma may arise from an existing mole (nevus) or spontaneously from previously normal skin. All new or changing moles need to be assessed to exclude malignancy.

and hepatic function should be monitored regularly

- Aberrations in the pituitary-adrenal axis or thyroid hormone levels are possible. Clinicians should monitor for fatigue, nausea, vomiting, orthostasis, and blurry vision at regular intervals

Treatment pearls

- Gastrointestinal side effects are the most common reason for dose or treatment limitations. Treatment options include supportive care, systemic corticosteroids, and intravenous rehydration depending on the severity. Perforation is possible, and the clinician should have a low threshold for imaging throughout the treatment course
- Prophylactic daily systemic corticosteroid use has not been shown to be helpful and is not recommended
- Unlike cytotoxic therapies, the response to ipilimumab cannot be monitored by tumor size alone. Instead, the Immune-related Response Criteria (IRRC) can be used to follow disease activity
- Clinical trials are in progress combining ipilimumab, pembrolizumab, and nivolumab with newer biologic therapies targeting other elements of the melanoma proliferation pathway. Future treatment regimens will include combinations of multiple anti-tumor biologic medications

SMALL MOLECULE INHIBITORS FOR MELANOMA

Dermatologic indications
- Vemurafenib is EMA, MHRA, and FDA approved for metastatic and locally advanced, unresectable BRAF V600E mutated melanoma. Patients should be tested for this mutation prior to starting therapy

Background

BRAF, a protein kinase involved in the MAPK pathway, is commonly mutated in melanoma as well as in several other malignancies, leading to unchecked growth.

A majority of these mutations in melanoma involve a glutamic acid substitution for valine (V600E). Vemurafenib is a protein kinase inhibitor that targets this mutation.

Dermatologic prescribing

- Vemurafenib is a tablet, taken as 960 mg twice daily. The dose should not be reduced below 480 mg twice daily

Cautions

- *Renal/hepatic:* mild to moderate renal or hepatic disease does not affect dosage, but severe baseline disease should warrant caution

- *Lactation/pregnancy:* women should use contraception while on vemurafenib, and lactation is not recommended during its use

Common problems

- The most common side effects are hepatotoxicity, QT prolongation, fatigue, nausea, vomiting, and arthralgias. Frequent EKG monitoring and serially drawn hepatic panels are mandatory

- Photosensitivity is common, and patients should be told to photoprotect, particularly from UVA radiation. Both UV and radiation recall can occur

- Squamous cell carcinomas, keratoacanthomas, and verrucous keratoses occur frequently, and may require cryotherapy, intralesional treatment, or even surgical excision for advanced cases. These often occur within the first few months of therapy, but are usually not dose limiting

- Melanoma (wild type BRAF) has also been reported, and any baseline melanocytic lesions in patients on vemurafenib should be frequently monitored with a low threshold for biopsy

- Palmo-plantar hyperkeratosis develops over friction and pressure prone sites. Severe sloughing can occur. Preventive measures are often necessary, such as following with podiatry and use of special shoes or gloves. Topical corticosteroids can be used for treatment

- A generalized drug eruption is possible as well as seborrheic dermatitis, alopecia, a keratosis pilaris-like eruption, and panniculitis

Treatment pearls

- Concurrent treatment with ipilimumab has shown worsening side effect profiles, particularly hepatotoxicity and cutaneous eruptions

- Most cutaneous side effects occur in the early stages of treatment. Close dermatology follow-up during this period is essential

- Those with prior sun damage are particularly prone to cutaneous reactions. Patients should be reminded that direct sunlight is not necessary for phototoxicity. Even activities such as driving can result in sufficient UV exposure to cause a reaction

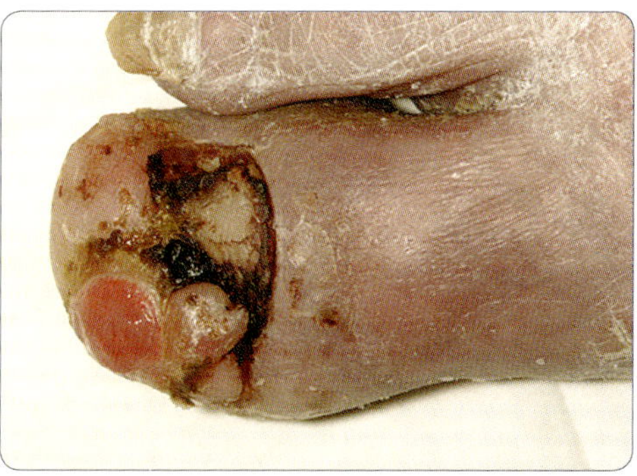

Figure 35.2 Amelanotic melanoma of the toe. Late stage melanomas with metastasis are increasingly treated with biologic therapies.

SMALL MOLECULE INHIBITORS FOR BASAL CELL CARCINOMA

Dermatologic indications

- Vismodegib is the only approved agent for locally advanced and metastatic basal cell carcinoma (BCC)

Background

Vismodegib is a small molecule inhibitor of Smoothened (SMO), a signalling protein in the sonic hedgehog pathway (SHH). This pathway is aberrant in most cases of BCC.

PTCH-1 is a protein that usually serves to check the activity of SMO and undergoes a loss of function mutation in BCC. Vismodegib inhibits SMO, thereby preventing growth.

Dermatologic prescribing

- Vismodegib is taken as a tablet, 150 mg daily

Cautions

- *Hepatic/renal:* there are no recommendations for dose alteration with baseline hepatic or renal disease

- *Pregnancy/lactation:* given the sonic hedgehog pathway's pivotal role in embryogenesis, vismodegib is potently teratogenic, and pregnancy is absolutely contraindicated. Women and men must use contraception while on vismodegib. Lactation is also not recommended

Common problems

- Fatigue and weight loss are commonly seen

- There have been case reports of SCC and keratoacanthoma developing while on vismodegib, and this is under investigation

- *Muscle spasms:* the most frequent side effect resulting in treatment discontinuation. Creatine kinase (CK) levels should be monitored

- *Dysgeusia:* the SHH pathway is essential in the development of tongue papillae that function in taste

- *Alopecia:* usually Grade 2. Topical minoxidil can be used throughout therapy with limited effectiveness

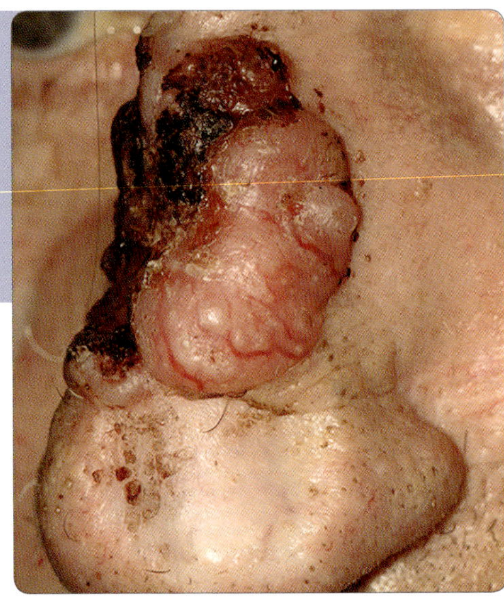

Figure 35.3 Basal cell carcinoma at nasal bridge. Vismodegib may be used to treat inoperable tumours or to reduce tumour size prior to surgery.

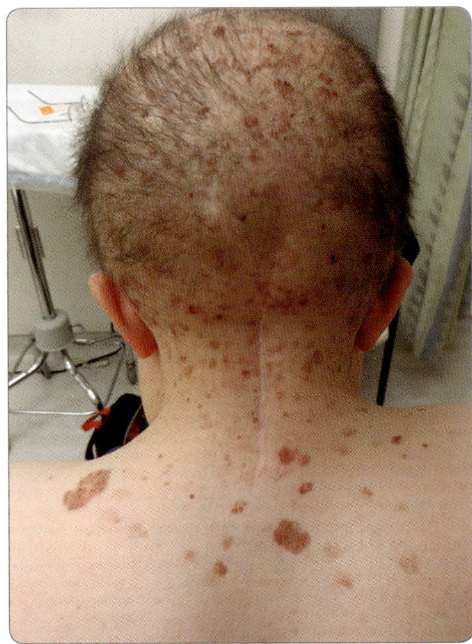

Figure 35.4 A teenager with basal cell nevus syndrome (Gorlin syndrome) who was subsequently treated with vismodegib. Courtesy of Dr Chrys Schmults, Brigham and Women's Hospital, Boston, USA.

Treatment pearls

- Almost every patient treated with vismodegib will experience a side effect. Breaks between dosing may be necessary to improve the tolerability of treatment
- Vismodegib may be of particular benefit to patients with Gorlin syndrome
- Patients with alopecia due to vismodegib can expect reversal after treatment cessation. If used, minoxidil should be continued 6 months after stopping vismodegib
- Patients should be advised to eliminate other causes of dysgeusia by maintaining consistent oral hygiene, controlling baseline esophageal reflux, and treating post nasal drip
- Muscle relaxants, such as cyclobenzaprine, can be prescribed for patients with muscle spasms

Further reading

Chapman PB, Hauschild A, Robert C, et al. Improved survival with vemurafenib in melanoma with BRAF V600E mutation. N Engl J Med 2011; 364:2507–2516.

Hodi SF, O'Day SJ, McDermott DF, et al. Improved survival with ipilimumab in patients with metastatic melanoma. N Engl J Med 2010; 363:711–723.

Iarrobino A, Messina JL, Kudchadkar R, et al. Emergence of a squamous cell carcinoma phenotype following treatment of metastatic basal cell carcinoma with vismodegib. J Am Acad Dermatol 2013; 69:e33–34.

Macdonald JB, Macdonald B, Golitz LE, et al. Cutaneous adverse effects of targeted therapies: Part II: Inhibitors of intracellular molecular signaling pathways. J Am Dermatol 2015; 72:221–236.

Sekulic A, Migden MR, Oro AE, et al. Efficacy and safety of vismodegib in advanced basal-cell carcinoma. N Engl J Med 2012; 366:2171–2179.

Weber, JS, Kähler KC, Hauschild A. Management of immune-related adverse events and kinetics of response with ipilimumab. J Clin Oncol 2012; 30:2691–2697.

Wolchok JD, Hoos A, O'Day S, et al. Guidelines for the evaluation of immune therapy activity in solid tumors: immune-related response criteria. Clin Cancer Res 2009; 15: 7412–7420.

Biologic therapy: rituximab

Dermatologic indications

- Off label use for autoimmune bullous disease, especially pemphigus vulgaris, is common. Some studies have also looked at its use in chronic graft versus host disease

- *Other uses:* mucous membrane pemphigoid, epidermolysis bullosa acquisita (EBA), vasculitis, cutaneous involvement in systemic sclerosis, dermatomyositis

- *Licensed indications:* include CD20-positive non-Hodgkin's lymphoma, CD20-positive diffuse large B-cell non-Hodgkin's lymphoma, CD20-positive chronic lymphocytic leukemia, rheumatoid arthritis, granulomatosis with polyangiitis (GPA) (Wegener's granulomatosis), microscopic polyangiitis (MPA)

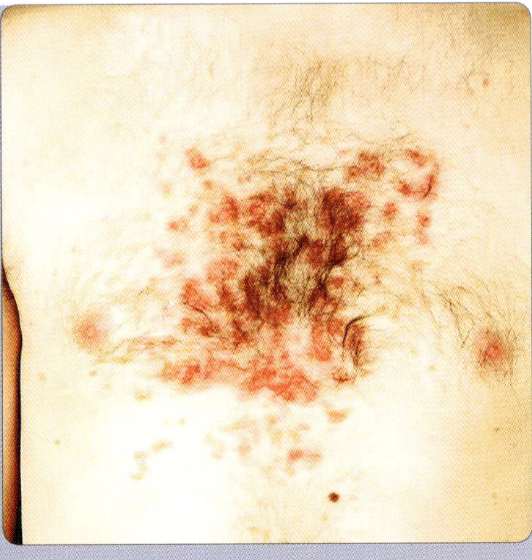

Figure 36.1 Pemphigus vulgaris with superficial bullae and erosions on the chest.

Background

Rituximab is an engineered chimeric monoclonal antibody that binds to CD20, an antigen found on pre-B cells and mature B cells.

Dermatologic prescribing

- There are two main approaches to dosing protocols, which have both been used for dermatologic indications. Both are often, but not always, supplemented by corticosteroids, other immunosuppressive agents, and/or IVIG. Selection of a particular regimen is clinician-dependent

- The regimen historically used for lymphomas involves intravenous infusion of 375 mg/m^2 BSA weekly for four doses

- The regimen classically used for treating autoimmune diseases, such as rheumatoid arthritis, involves 500 mg or 1000 mg (most often 1000 mg) intravenous infusion on days 1 and 15 of the cycle

- Repetition of the cycles may occur depending on clinical response or relapse. A typical interval between cycles is approximately 6 months

- Rituximab has been shown to induce remission in cases of severe pemphigus vulgaris resistant to other standard immunosuppressive regimens. The overall rate of side effects may be lower than traditional treatment combinations, which include high doses of systemic corticosteroids. Further studies are needed to clarify the precise role of rituximab in pemphigus therapy

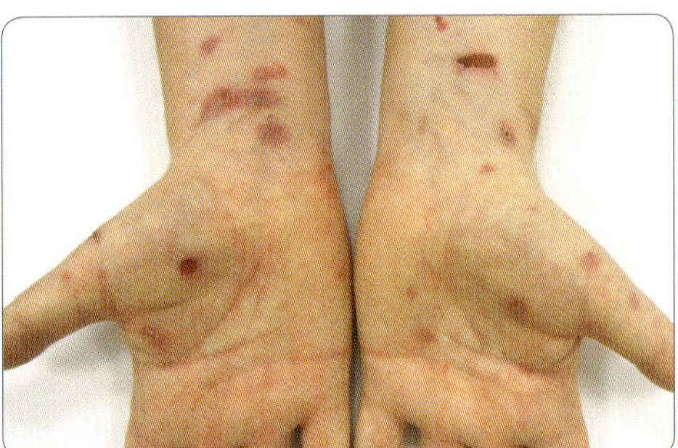

Figure 36.2 Scarring on both wrists following bullae from epidermolysis bullosa acquisita (EBA) treated with rituximab.

- Rituximab has also shown promising results in treating mucous membrane pemphigoid and epidermolysis bullosa acquisita (EBA)

Cautions

- As with other forms of biologic immunosupression a full infection screen is required prior to commencing treatment. This needs to include testing for TB, HIV and viral hepatitis. Varicella serology is also often checked to confirm immunity to chickenpox

- *Renal/hepatic:* there is no known contraindication with baseline renal or hepatic impairment

- *Pregnancy/lactation:* women should use contraception and avoid pregnancy while taking rituximab. Breast feeding is not recommended

Common problems

- Rituximab is generally very well tolerated

- Infusion reactions are most commonly seen with the first administered dose of rituximab. Patients can experience rigors, fevers, and even angioedema in severe cases. All patients given rituximab are premedicated with a dose of intravenous glucocorticoids

- Progressive multifocal leukoencephalopathy is a very rare but fatal complication

- Mucocutaneous eruptions are rarely observed

- Hepatitis B reactivation is a very serious concern. All patients should be tested with a hepatitis panel to check for quiescent active infection or cleared prior infection prior to treatment with rituximab

- Patients on rituximab are at an increased risk of infection given the suppression of both B cells and immunoglobulins, particularly IgM

- Post treatment prolonged hypogammaglobulinaemia is a rare complication and may require supplementation with replacement doses of intravenous immunoglobulin

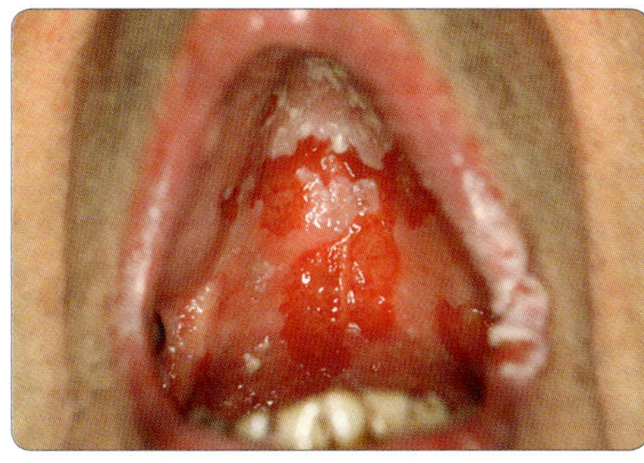

Figure 36.3 Pemphigus vulgaris often presents with oral involvement.

Further reading

Ahmed AR, Shetty S. A comprehensive analysis of treatment outcomes in patients with pemphigus vulgaris treated with rituximab. Autoimmun Rev 2015; 14:323–331.

Ahmed AR, Spigelman Z, Cavacini L, Posner MR. Treatment of pemphigus vulgaris with rituximab and intravenous immune globulin. N Engl J Med 2006; 355:1772–1779.

Cutler C, Miklos D, Kim HT, et al. Rituximab for steroid-refractory chronic graft-versus-host disease. Blood 2015; 108:756–762.

Dinh HV, McCormack C, Hall S, Prince HM. Rituximab for the treatment of the skin manifestations of dermatomyositis: a report of 3 cases. J Am Acad Dermatol 2007; 56:148–153.

Treatment pearls

- A PPD or interferon gamma release assay should be ordered to rule out latent tuberculosis before starting rituximab

- A hepatitis panel should be performed on every patient prior to treatment initiation. Check a hepatitis B surface antigen and hepatitis B core antibody to rule out chronic or acute hepatitis B infection. A hepatitis B surface antibody can be checked to ensure prior vaccination. It is also advisable to check a hepatitis C antibody

- HIV status should be checked prior to treatment initiation

- Patients should not receive live vaccines while on rituximab, including the varicella zoster vaccine. They should be up to date on all recommended vaccines, including hepatitis B, pneumococcal, tetanus, and influenza prior to starting therapy

- Serious reactions to rituximab typically occur during the first dose. However, most centers still pre-medicate before every dose of rituximab with intravenous methylprednisolone and intravenous or oral diphenhydramine or an alternate antihistamine

- Improvements in immunobullous diseases will generally be apparent within 2-4 weeks. Other immunosuppressive therapies should be reduced soon after rituximab treatment

- Following rituximab treatment for pemphigus, most patients will remain on low doses of standard immunosuppression. This is believed to increase the interval before needing further rituximab

Colchicine

Dermatologic indications

- Behçet's disease (particularly effective for oral and genital aphthosis and joint symptoms)
- Sweet's syndrome, pyoderma gangrenosum, leukocytoclastic vasculitis, urticarial vasculitis, recurrent aphthous stomatitis
- *Also used for:* autoimmune bullous diseases (epidermolysis bullosa acquisita, IgA pemphigus, linear IgA bullous dermatosis), relapsing polychondritis, chronic urticaria, dystrophic calcinosis cutis, autoinflammatory syndromes, acute gout flares, familial Mediterranean fever (FMF)

Background

Colchicine is an alkaloid derived from a plant, *Colchicum autumnale*. It has both anti-mitotic and anti-inflammatory properties, mediated primarily by binding tubulin and inhibiting microtubule polymerization.

It blocks mitosis in metaphase, thus causing greater toxicity to tissues with rapid cell turnover such as gastrointestinal mucosa and bone marrow.

It concentrates in leukocytes, particularly neutrophils, and exerts an anti-inflammatory effect by interfering with neutrophil migration, degranulation, and phagocytosis.

Mean oral bioavailability in healthy individuals is 45%, but this is highly variable, resulting in varied individual responses to the same dose.

Peak plasma concentrations occur 1 hour after administration, with maximal anti-inflammatory effects developing over 24–48 hours.

It is metabolized in the liver and mainly eliminated by biliary excretion. A small amount, 10–20%, is eliminated unchanged in the urine.

Dermatologic prescribing

- *Route:* oral. Injection has not been approved by the US Food and Drug Administration (FDA)
- *Dose:* 0.5–0.6 mg two to three times daily. The drug must be shielded from UV light to prevent degradation into inactive products. The dose can subsequently be tapered to the minimally effective dose for disease after a period of response

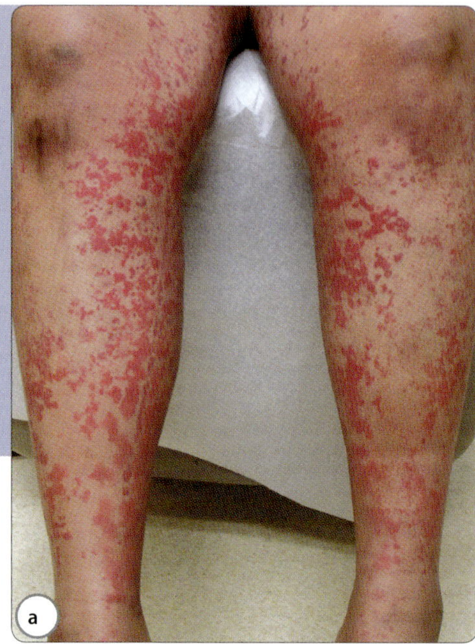

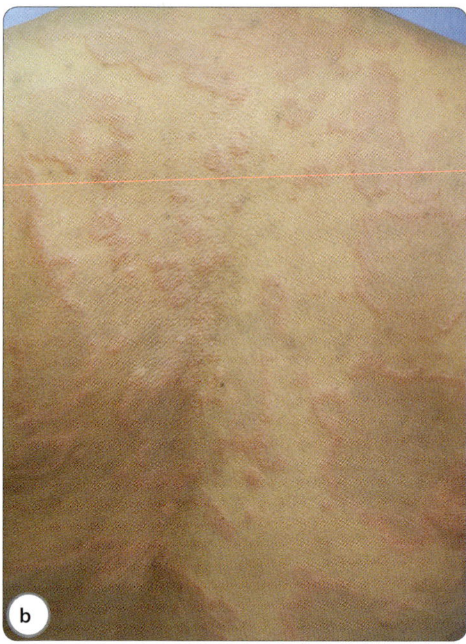

Figure 37.1 (a) Leukocytoclastic vasculitis: symmetrically distributed palpable purpura on the bilateral lower extremities; (b) Urticarial vasculitis: annular and polycyclic erythematous urticarial plaques with dusky centers.

- Monitoring of complete blood counts (CBC), renal and liver function, and urinalysis should be performed before the initiation of therapy and every 3 months thereafter; monthly laboratory monitoring for the first few months of therapy may also be considered

Cautions

- Prior hypersensitivity reaction
- Blood dyscrasias
- Severe renal, hepatic, gastrointestinal, or cardiac disease
- *Medical interactions:* CYP3A4 and P-glycoprotein inhibitors, such as clarithromycin, erythromycin, ketoconazole, cyclosporine, and grapefruit juice, can increase colchicine concentrations. Co-administration with statins may increase the risk of myopathy
- *Pregnancy/lactation risk:* contraindicated in pregnancy. It should be used with caution during lactation as it is excreted into breast milk although no adverse outcomes have been observed in colchicine-exposed breastfed infants

Common problems

- *Most common:* gastrointestinal symptoms (diarrhea, abdominal pain, nausea, vomiting), especially at doses of 0.5–0.6 mg administered three times daily. These side effects are usually mild and dose-dependent, and may resolve with dose reduction
- While colchicine is generally well-tolerated at therapeutic doses, doses of 0.5–0.8 mg/kg/day are considered highly toxic, and doses of more than 0.8 mg/kg/day may be lethal
- *Acute overdose:* gastrointestinal symptoms within 24 hours of ingestion, and multiple organ failure within seven days. Treatment is usually supportive
- *Chronic overdose:* typically occurs if the dose is not adjusted for renal dysfunction or presence of concomitant interacting medications. Symptoms include peripheral neuropathy, myopathy, bone marrow suppression, and alopecia; these usually resolve upon discontinuation of the drug

Treatment pearls

- Diarrhea is the most common gastrointestinal side effect, which occurs in 5–10% of individuals. This is in part due to increased peristaltic activity and may be controlled with aluminum containing antacids or antidiarrheal medications such as loperamide
- Tolerance may be improved by starting once-daily dosing and gradually increasing the frequency over a number of weeks. However, if symptoms of intolerance occur, discontinuing the medication to avoid more serious toxicity should be considered
- Individuals with mild to moderate hepatic and/or renal dysfunction must be closely monitored for adverse effects, and their dose should be reduced accordingly
- In renal dysfunction, the daily dose of colchicine should be adjusted according to the glomerular filtration rate (GFR). Suggested guidelines are as follows:
  - GFR 30–60 mL/min, daily dose should be reduced to 0.6 mg once daily
  - GFR 15–30 mL/min, daily dose should be reduced to 0.6 mg every 2–3 days
  - GFR <15 mL/min or on hemodialysis, avoid use
- Colchicine should be used with caution in the elderly. Some studies suggest that the daily dose should be reduced by 50% in patients >70 years of age

Further reading

Cocco G, Chu DC, Pandolfi S. Colchicine in clinical medicine. A guide for internists. Eur J Intern Med 2010; 21:503–508.

Davis LS, LeBlanc KG, Knable AL, Owen CE. Miscellaneous systemic drugs. In: Wolverton SE (Ed). Comprehensive Dermatologic Therapy, 3rd Edn. Philadelphia: Elsevier-Saunders, 2012.

Niel E, Scherrmann JM. Colchicine today. Joint Bone Spine 2006; 73:672–678.

Slobodnick A, Shah B, Pillinger MH, Krasnokutsky S. Colchicine: old and new. Am J Med 2014; 128:461–470.

Sullivan TP, King LE Jr, Boyd AS. Colchicine in dermatology. J Am Acad Dermatol 1998; 39:993–999.

Cyclophosphamide

Dermatologic indications

- Advanced cutaneous T-cell lymphoma (mycosis fungoides), immunobullous disorders (e.g. pemphigus vulgaris, bullous pemphigoid, and mucous membrane pemphigoid)

- Also used in autoimmune disorders including vasculitis (e.g. granulomatosis with polyangiitis), systemic lupus erythematosus, Behçet's disease, and pyoderma gangrenosum

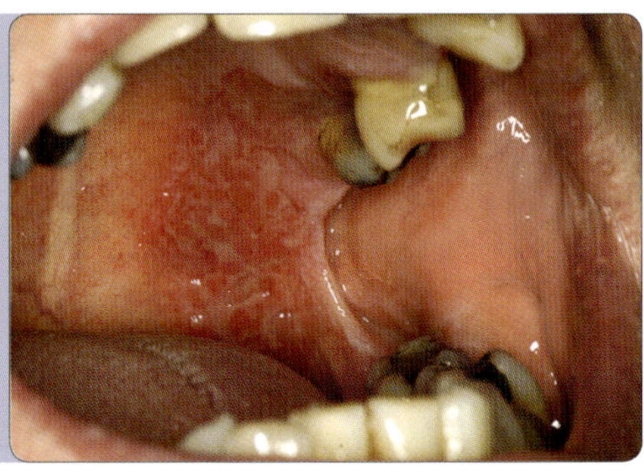

Figure 38.1 Intraoral mucous membrane pemphigoid.

Background

Cyclophosphamide is an alkylating agent that selectively inhibits proliferation, differentiation, and activity of B lymphocytes.

It is metabolized by cytochrome P450 in the liver to active metabolites, mainly phosphoramide mustard and acrolein; both cyclophosphamide and its metabolites are excreted in the urine.

Cyclophosphamide is available in intravenous and oral formulations. It is well-absorbed when given orally.

When cyclophosphamide is used for dermatologic indications, it is generally given in a lower dose than when used in oncology.

Strict monitoring is required during treatment, and the duration of therapy depends on clinical improvement.

Dermatologic prescribing

- *Oral:* 50–150 mg daily

- *Intravenous:* intermittent infusions of 100–500 mg every 2–4 weeks

- Pulsed intravenous cyclophosphamide is co-prescribed with:

- Anti-emetics such as domperidone

- Mesna, a sulfhydryl donor binds acrolein to prevent sterile haemorrhagic cystitis. Mesna doses are typically 200 mg 30 minutes before, 2 hours after, and 6 hours after cyclophosphamide

- Consider adding IV dexamethasone 100 mg or methylprednisolone 1 g daily for 3 days (see Treatment pearls on following page)

- Screening blood tests including a complete blood count, renal function, urinalysis, and liver function as well as hepatitis serologies and HIV testing are warranted

- At each infusion, a complete blood count, renal function tests, electrolyte levels, urinalysis, and a clinical assessment should be undertaken

- Clinical assessment should include a review of temperature, history of new signs/symptoms of infection, disease status, consideration of how previous doses were tolerated, and doses of other immunosuppressive medications prescribed. Treatment is contraindicated if there is evidence of concomitant active sepsis

Cautions

- Acute porphyrias, diabetes mellitus, previous or concurrent mediastinal irradiation (risk of cardiotoxicity)

- Pregnancy: cyclophosphamide is teratogenic and should not be used in pregnancy. Pregnancy must be avoided for at least 6 weeks following treatment

- Fertility: cyclophosphamide increases the risk of gonadal failure in both sexes and its use should be carefully considered in patients of reproductive age

- Secondary malignancies have developed in some patients previously treated with cyclophosphamide, most frequently transitional cell carcinoma of the bladder and myeloproliferative or lymphoproliferative disorders

- Interactions: myelosuppression may occur when cyclophosphamide is given concurrently with allopurinol; barbiturates enhance the metabolism of cyclophosphamide to active alkylating agents

Common problems

- Anorexia and nausea are common and typically improve with anti-emetics

- Dose adjustment may be required in the setting of:

- Hepatic impairment (e.g. transaminases or alkaline phosphatase more than two to three times the upper limit of normal)

- Renal impairment (decreased renal excretion may result in increased plasma levels of cyclophosphamide and its metabolites)

- Hematologic abnormalities or toxicity

- Additive toxicity may occur if cyclophosphamide is given in combination with other cytotoxic or immunosuppressive drugs

Further reading

Ahmed AR, Hombal SM. Cyclophosphamide (Cytoxan): A review on relevant pharmacology and clinical uses. J Am Acad Dermatol 1984; 11:1115–1126.

Gual A, Iranzo P, Mascaró JM Jr. Treatment of bullous pemphigoid with low-dose oral cyclophosphamide: a case series of 20 patients. J Eur Acad Dermatol Venereol 2014; 28:814–818.

Pasricha JS, Ramji G. Pulse therapy with dexamethasone–cyclophosphamide in pemphigus. Indian J Dermatol Venereol Leprol 1984; 50:199-203.

Pasricha JS. Current regimen of pulse therapy for pemphigus: minor modifications, improved results. Indian J Dermatol Venereol Leprol 2008; 74:217-21.

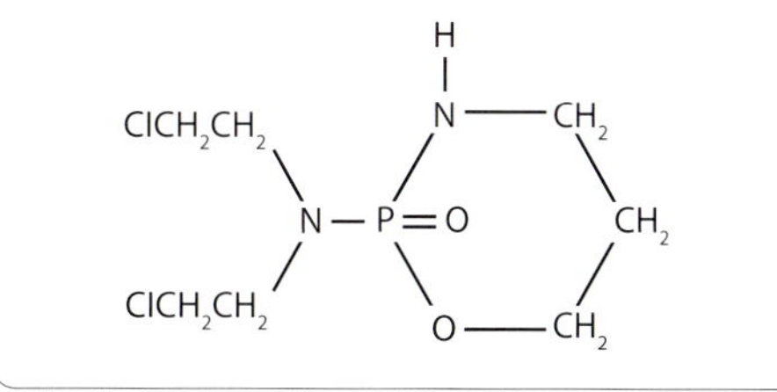

Figure 38.2 Molecular structure of cyclophosphamide.

Treatment pearls

- Varicella immunity should be established and unprotected individuals vaccinated pre-treatment

- Higher doses of cyclophosphamide are commonly associated with varicella zoster (shingles). Booster vaccinations, lowering of cyclophosphamide dose, and rapid initiation of antiviral treatment is important

- Daily oral cyclophosphamide provides significant immunosuppression and results in a high cumulative dose. Therefore, many centers use oral cyclophosphamide in pulsed regimens (e.g. weekly) in order to reduce the risk of adverse effects while still maintaining efficacy

- There is now considerable evidence demonstrating the efficacy of cyclophosphamide in conjunction with either oral or intravenous corticosteroids in pemphigus vulgaris. A series of 300 patients with pemphigus were treated with monthly intravenous cyclophosphamide and dexamethasone pulse therapy together with oral cyclophosphamide between pulses. 190 patients (63%) achieved complete remission, 123 (41%) of these for more than 2 years and 48 (16%) for more than 5 years. An additional study of 50 patients with pemphigus reported cyclophosphamide and dexamethasone pulse therapy to be effective in 88% of patients

- Cyclophosphamide has also been used in the treatment of pemphigoid and its variants. In one study, thirteen patients with severe refractory mucous membrane pemphigoid treated with oral cyclophosphamide (2 mg/kg) without corticosteroids showed an overall response rate of 69%, with a median time to disease control of 8 weeks (range 4–52 weeks). A retrospective case series of 20 patients with refractory bullous pemphigoid showed that low dose oral cyclophosphamide (50–100 mg) led to a complete response in 11 (58%) patients and clinical remission in 8 (40%) patients

Dermatologic indications

- Psoriasis, atopic dermatitis, pyoderma gangrenosum
- *Also commonly used for:* dyshidrotic eczema, chronic urticaria, solar urticaria, Behçet disease, pityriasis rubra pilaris, dermatomyositis, pemphigus vulgaris, epidermolysis bullosa acquisita, lichen planus, chronic actinic dermatitis, polymorphic light eruption, lichen planus, lichen planopilaris, prurigo nodularis, alopecia areata, Hailey–Hailey disease, eosinophilic pustular folliculitis, hidradenitis suppurativa, Stevens–Johnson syndrome, toxic epidermal necrolysis

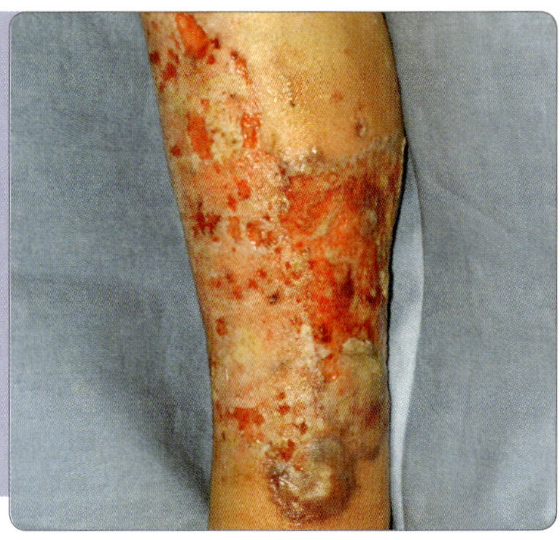

Figure 39.1 Pyoderma gangrenosum in the setting of inflammatory bowel disease.

Background

Cyclosporine forms a complex with cyclophilin which inactivates calcineurin phosphorylase, preventing the phosphorylation of nuclear factor of activated T-cells (NFAT) and, therefore, inhibits the transcription of interleukin-2. Interleukin 2 is needed for full activation of the T-cell pathway.

Dermatologic prescribing

- Screen for hypertension, HIV, and viral hepatitis prior to initiation. Check renal function, liver function, complete blood count, serum magnesium, potassium, uric acid, lipid profile
- Monitoring should occur every 2 weeks for the first 3 months then monthly thereafter. Increase the frequency of monitoring with dose adjustment or co-administration of NSAIDs
- Dosing is by ideal body weight:
  - *Initial dose:* 2–5 mg/kg/day, divided twice daily (disease dependent)
  - *Titration:* increase by 0.5 mg/kg/day if insufficient response is seen after 4 weeks of treatment. Additional dosage increases may be made every 2 weeks if needed. Dose reductions are necessary if the serum creatinine increases
  - *Maximum dose:* 5 mg/kg/day
  - *Route:* oral, also available in intravenous form
- Discontinue if no benefit is seen by 12 weeks of therapy at the maximum dose
- Short-term interval therapy: treatment is continued until substantial improvement of the skin disease has occurred. Subsequently, the dose is tapered and discontinued, and treatment is continued with another medication. In the event of a relapse of cutaneous disease, cyclosporine therapy can be reinitiated
- Long-term therapy: chronic and/or severe skin diseases with a strong tendency to recur can be treated with long-term cyclosporine therapy. In this case, it is imperative that the lowest possible dose is used. Regular determination of blood pressure and of renal function parameters is of critical importance. With long-term therapy, elevation of serum creatinine by >30% can be expected in up to 50% of patients. This is usually dose-dependent and reversible upon discontinuation. Elevation in the serum creatinine should lead to cyclosporine dose-reduction. After therapy for a maximum of 1–2 years, an attempt at discontinuation should be made.

Cautions

- Cyclosporine is contraindicated in those with uncontrolled hypertension or infection. Current or prior malignancy, except for basal cell carcinoma, is often considered a contraindication
- *Liver disease:* cyclosporine has extensive hepatic metabolism, and exposure is increased in hepatic impairment. Monitoring and dose reduction is recommended
- *Renal disease:* cyclosporine should generally be avoided in renal impairment as the medication can exacerbate renal disease. Elevations in serum creatinine should prompt a dose-reduction
- *Interactions:* cyclosporine has multiple potential drug interactions which should be assessed in all patients. Statins, calcium channel blockers, loop diuretics, macrolide antibiotics, tetracycline antibiotics, azole antifungal agents, methotrexate, corticosteroids, mycophenolate mofetil, and NSAIDs are common drugs that interact with cyclosporine
- *Pregnancy/lactation risk:* risk in pregnancy cannot be ruled out. Cyclosporine should be

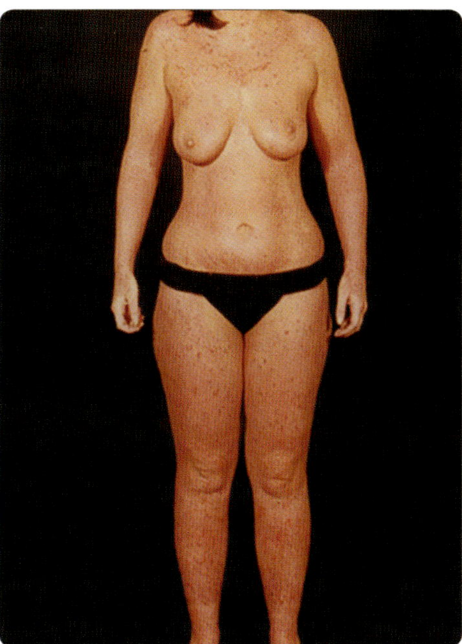

Figure 39.2 Generalized severe atopic dermatitis in early adulthood.

avoided in the first trimester. It enters breast milk and is not recommended with breast feeding

- *Prior PUVA:* cyclosporine should be avoided in those with a high cumulative dose of previous psoralen and UVA light phototherapy (PUVA) as this can increase the risk of cutaneous malignancy

Common problems

- *Hypertension:* risk is higher with increasing dose or duration of treatment

- *Infections:* immunosuppression raises the risk of fatal bacterial, viral, fungal, and protozoal infections (including opportunistic infections)

- *Malignancy:* there is an increased risk of lymphomas and skin cancers. Patients should practice careful photoprotection

- *Nephrotoxicity:* the risk is increased with increasing doses, especially doses >5 mg/kg/day, and duration, particularly >2 years. Monitor renal function closely

- *Hepatotoxicity:* liver injury (cholestasis, jaundice, hepatitis, liver failure) can occur with cyclosporine use. Co-administration with other hepatotoxic medications should be avoided. Improves with dose reduction

- *Gingival hyperplasia:* occurs more frequently with concomitant nifedipine use. Intensive oral hygiene, particularly plaque control, is helpful in preventing and treating this. Gingival surgery may be required if treatment is continued

- *Cutaneous side effects:* hypertrichosis (60%), epidermal cysts (28%), keratosis pilaris (21%), acne (15%), folliculitis (12%), and sebaceous hyperplasia (10%)

- *Tremor:* is common with long-term use

Further reading

Amor KT, Ryan C, Menter A. The use of cyclosporine in dermatology: part I. J Am Acad Dermatol 2010; 63:925–946.

Mrowietz U1, Klein CE, Reich K, et al. Cyclosporine therapy in dermatology. J Dtsch Dermatol Ges 2009; 7:474–479.

Ryan C, Amor KT, Menter A. The use of cyclosporine in dermatology: part II. J Am Acad Dermatol 2010; 63:949–972.

Treatment pearls

- Vaccination should take place before the initiation of treatment. Live vaccines are contraindicated while on cyclosporine, and immune response to inactivated vaccines may be diminished

- In most cases, cyclosporine should be used primarily for induction therapy (for up to 6–12 months) due to its rapid effects. On the basis of the safety profile, its use as a long-term therapy is only indicated in exceptional cases

- Combination with topical products is advisable as the dose of cyclosporine can often be reduced

- Cyclosporine should not be combined with phototherapy, photochemotherapy, or acitretin

- If hypertension develops, the first step is to initiate antihypertensive therapy (recommended: amlodipine, isradipine; avoid: nifedipine, verapamil, diltiazem). Then dose reduction should be considered thereafter

- Development of renal impairment: elevation of serum creatinine by at least 30% over the individual baseline on two successive blood samples at 2 weeks apart is sufficient to require a dose reduction by 25% for at least 4 weeks

- If there is no improvement after 4 weeks of dose reduction, cyclosporine should be discontinued

Dapsone and sulfapyridine

Dermatologic indications

- *Dapsone (systemic):* dermatitis herpetiformis, leprosy
- *Dapsone (topical):* acne vulgaris
- *Sulfapyridine:* dermatitis herpetiformis
- *Also used for:* linear IgA bullous dermatosis, erythema elevatum diutinum, bullous lupus erythematosus, leukocytoclastic vasculitis, urticarial vasculitis, IgA pemphigus, bullous pemphigoid, pyoderma gangrenosum, Sweet's syndrome, chronic idiopathic urticaria, Behçet's disease

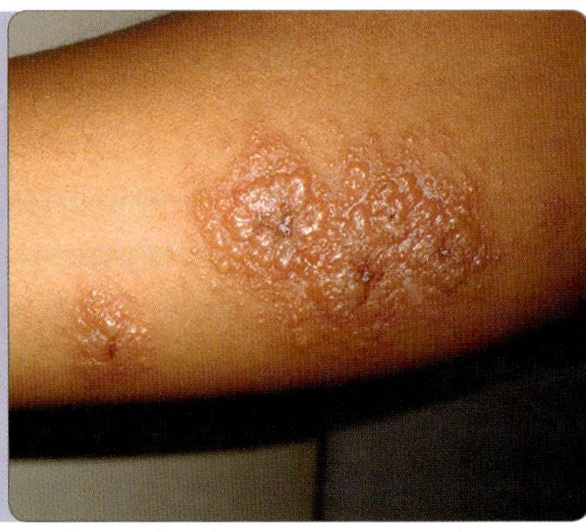

Figure 40.1 Annular and 'cluster of jewels' arrangement of tense bullae characteristic of linear IgA bullous dermatosis.

Background

Dapsone and sulfapyridine are antimicrobials that disrupt folic acid synthesis by inhibiting dihydropteroate synthetase. Dapsone's antimicrobial effects are responsible for its efficacy in treating leprosy.

Dapsone and sulfapyridine also inhibit neutrophil chemotaxis and the neutrophil respiratory burst (via inhibition of neutrophil myeloperoxidase), and these anti-neutrophilic effects are responsible for their effectiveness in treating neutrophilic dermatoses. Dapsone additionally inhibits eosinophil myeloperoxidase, making it potentially useful in eosinophil driven dermatoses.

A hydroxylated metabolite of dapsone is responsible for its hematologic side effects.

Dermatologic prescribing

Dapsone

- *Leprosy:* 100 mg once daily for 6–12 months. To prevent resistance, dapsone is not used as monotherapy when treating leprosy
- *Dermatitis herpetiformis (DH):* 50–200 mg daily. After control is achieved, titrate slowly to lowest effective dose
- *Neutrophilic dermatoses:* same dosing as for DH
- *Baseline laboratory tests:*
  - Glucose-6-phosphate dehydrogenase (G6PD) level, complete blood count (CBC) with differential, and liver and renal function tests
- *Monitoring laboratory tests:*
  - CBC with differential (initially requires close monitoring (every 2–4 weeks), then every 3 months thereafter. A reticulocyte count may be helpful if significant anemia is noted. Checking a methemoglobin level is indicated if the patient has evidence of excessive fatigue, headaches, or other cardiopulmonary symptoms. Liver function should be monitored every 2–4 weeks initially and then every 3 months. Renal function should be monitored every 3 months

Sulfapyridine

- *Dermatitis herpetiformis:* 1–4 g daily (start with a low dose such as 500 mg three times daily and increase as tolerated)
- Monitoring as for dapsone

Cautions

- *G6PD deficiency:* risk of massive hemolysis. Contraindicated in patients with G6PD deficiency
- *Liver or renal disease:* hepatic and renal excretion. Use alternative drug or reduced dose with careful monitoring
- *Pre-existing peripheral neuropathy:* is a relative contraindication
- *Medication interactions:* avoid use of folate antagonists including sulfonamide antibiotics and methotrexate. If concomitant methotrexate is required, consider using a reduced dose and careful laboratory monitoring. Antimalarials and prilocaine may increase the risk of hemolysis and methemoglobinemia
- *Pregnancy/lactation risk:* avoid during pregnancy. In addition, dapsone is excreted in breast milk and may cause neonatal hemolysis. Pregnancy/lactation safety data for sulfapyridine is limited. Sulfapyridine may cause reversible oligospermia

Common problems

- Hematologic side effects:
  - Hemolysis is dose dependent and may occur in all patients on dapsone. Symptomatic anemia or rapidly falling hemoglobin levels may be

managed with dose reductions. Refractory anemia may necessitate discontinuation. Sulfapyridine uncommonly causes hemolysis

- Methemoglobinemia typically presents as fatigue, dyspnea, headaches, and cyanosis. Severe methemoglobinemia may cause fatal cardiac arrhythmias. Severe cases should be treated with methylene blue 100–300 mg daily (contraindicated in G6PD deficiency) or plasma exchange

- Agranulocytosis is an idiosyncratic, potentially fatal complication of treatment and should be suspected in any patient with flu-like symptoms or unexplainable fever

- Peripheral neuropathy (distal motor rather than sensory) is more common with dapsone than with sulfapyridine

- Dapsone hypersensitivity syndrome may present with a cutaneous eruption, elevated liver function tests, eosinophilia, and lymphadenopathy

Further reading

Edhegard K, Russel PH III. Dapsone. In: Wolverton SE (Ed) Comprehensive Dermatologic Drug Therapy. Philadelphia: Elsevier Health Sciences, 2012.

Lorincz AL, Pearson RW. Sulfapyridine and sulphone type drugs in dermatology. Arch Dermatol 1962; 85:2–16.

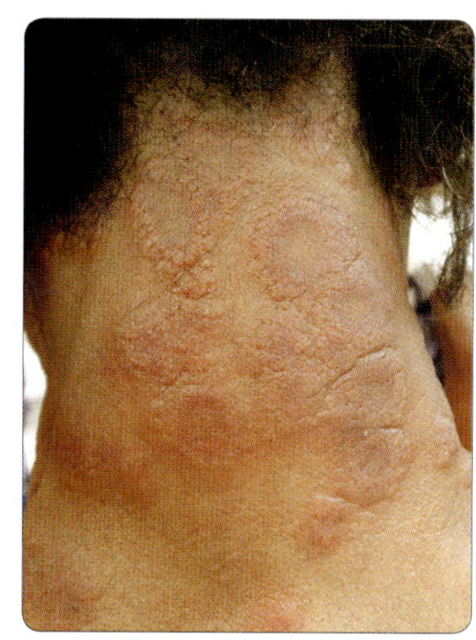

Figure 40.2 Sweet's syndrome. Edematous, tender plaques affecting the head and neck of a woman with breast cancer.

Swartzentruber GS, Yanta JH, Pizon AF. Methemoglobinemia as a complication of topical dapsone. N Engl J Med 2015; 372:491–492.

Treatment pearls

- When considering therapy with dapsone, it is important to adequately assess the patient prior to initiation. A complete history should be obtained in all patients, including screening for underlying cardiopulmonary, renal, or hepatic dysfunction

- Dermatitis herpetiformis typically responds within 24–48 hours; this quick response may aid in the diagnosis of DH

- Macrocytosis may occur in patients on dapsone and typically represents reticulocytosis

- Hemolysis of aged erythrocytes may falsely lower the HbA1c level used for diabetes monitoring

- Prophylactic administration of vitamin E (800 IU daily) or cimetidine (400 mg three times daily) may decrease the risk of hemolysis and methemoglobinemia

- Methemoglobinemia has been reported in acne patients using topical dapsone

- When assessing for neuropathy, remember to assess for distal motor function. Asking about sensory function is less sensitive because the majority of patients present with motor impairment

- Photosensitivity has been reported with dapsone. Remember to counsel patients on sun avoidance/ protection

- Patients intolerant to dapsone may be treated with sulfasalazine 1–2 g daily. Sulfasalazine is metabolized into sulfapyridine and 5-ASA in the gut

- Sulfapyridine or sulfasalazine should be taken with water to prevent crystalluria with nephrolithiasis

- Severe reactions including toxic epidermal necrolysis and dapsone hypersensitivity syndrome are rare, but patients should be made aware of the warning signs and symptoms

Dermatologic indications

- Psoriasis
- *Also used for:* necrobiosis lipoidica diabeticorum, granuloma annulare

Background

Fumaric acid esters (FAEs) include monoethylfumarate (MMF) and dimethylfumarate (DMF). DMF is considered the active metabolite and is converted in the body into methyl hydrogen fumarate and then free fumaric acid.

There are several proposed mechanisms of action including a direct anti-inflammatory effect by downregulation of proinflammatory cytokines, inhibition of dendritic cell maturation, and a shift of T helper (Th) cells towards a Th-2 cytokine response, leading to inhibition of epidermal keratinocyte proliferation.

FAEs were first discovered by the German chemist Walter Schweckendiek in 1959 and have been commercially available since 1994 as Fumaderm (Biogen Idec GmbH), a mixture of dimethylfumarate with calcium, magnesium, and zinc salts of monoethylfumarate. However, fumaric acid esters are as yet unlicensed for the treatment of psoriasis in most countries other than Germany (e.g. the UK, USA, New Zealand).

Dermatologic prescribing

- Low and high strength preparations of Fumaderm are available, Fumaderm Initial and Fumaderm Full Strength respectively.

- The dose is gradually increased on a weekly basis

- Fumaderm Initial (30 mg DMF) once daily, increasing over 8 weeks up to a maximum dose of six Fumaderm Full Strength (120 mg DMF) as a divided dose of two tablets three times a day

- An example dosing scheme is given in **Table 41.1**

- The dose can slowly be tapered until the individual's maintenance dosage is reached

- Intermittent short course therapy or continuous maintenance treatment can be used

- Sudden cessation of therapy does not usually lead to rebound flaring of symptoms

- Clinical improvement is expected after approximately 6 weeks

- A 75% reduction in psoriasis area and severity index (PASI) is seen in 50–70% of patients after 16 weeks of treatment

Table 41.1 Example Fumaderm dosing scheme (adapted from Nast et al. 2012)

	Fumaderm initial (30 mg DMF): No. capsules am-midday-pm	Fumaderm (120 mg DMF) : No. capsules am-midday-pm
Week 1	1-0-0	
Week 2	1-0-1	
Week 3	1-1-1	
Week 4		1-0-0
Week 5		1-0-1
Week 6		1-1-1
Week 7		2-1-1
Week 8		2-1-2
Week 9		2-2-2

- Safe and effective longer term treatment has been reported. For example, a retrospective study of 249 patients treated with FAEs showed a mean length of treatment of 28 months (range 1 week to 106 months), with 26 patients (10%) maintained on very low dose FAEs (240 mg daily) for a mean treatment duration of 64 months (range 32–106 months)

- Regular monitoring of complete blood counts (CBC) and liver and renal function is recommended. German guidelines suggest

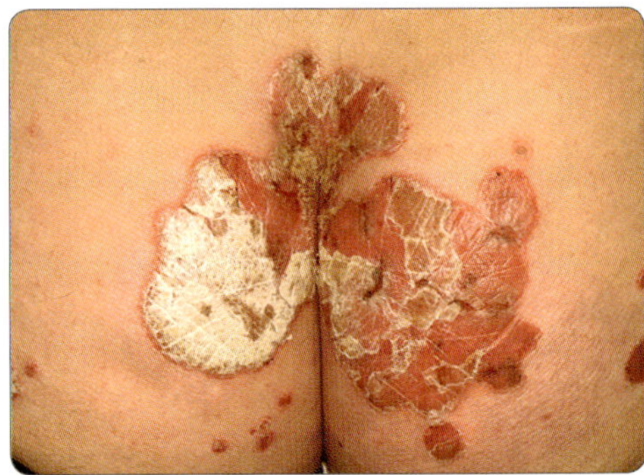

Figure 41.1 Chronic plaque psoriasis.

monthly CBC monitoring for the first four months and then every other month thereafter

- Proteinuria has been reported, and monitoring of the urine protein:creatinine ratio is advised

- Combination therapy with topical agents may be useful. There is evidence to support the use of FAEs with calcipotriol ointment. Concomitant use of other systemic drugs is not currently recommended

Cautions and common problems

- FAEs are contraindicated in patients with severe gastrointestinal disease, renal impairment, or hematologic disorders, and in pregnant and lactating women

- Gastrointestinal side effects such as nausea, bloating, or diarrhea are common and are experienced with varying degrees of severity by approximately two-thirds of patients, usually in the first few weeks of treatment

- Flushing is common at the outset of treatment in approximately one-third of patients

- Hematologic abnormalities including lymphocytopenia and eosinophilia are fairly common, although these are usually of no clinical significance and tend to resolve completely on treatment cessation

- Concomitant use with other immunosuppressive agents is not recommended

- Important: recent data suggest that the development of progressive multifocal leukoencephalopathy (PML) in association with FAE treatment is more common than previously recognized. Although still a rare complication, PML is currently untreatable. Some reports suggest that PML can arise without lymphocytopenia, suggesting that monitoring complete blood counts may be inadequate for prevention of this complication

Treatment pearls

- Slowly increasing the dose improves tolerability

- Gastrointestinal tolerability may be improved by taking tablets with milk

- Use of aspirin may improve the associated flushing, however, may make gastrointestinal side effects worse

- Measurement of lymphocyte subsets (CD4, CD8) is recommended if the lymphocyte count drops below 1×10^9/L. When the CD4 count is <200 cells/mm^3, prophylaxis against *Pneumocystis jiroveci* should be considered or the drug should be stopped

- The dose of FAEs should be halved if the lymphocyte count drops below 0.75×10^9/L

- FAEs should be stopped if the lymphocyte count drops below 0.5×10^9/L

- Dose reduction is also recommended if there is a persistent eosinophilia of ≥25% or a rise in serum creatinine of 30% above baseline

Further reading

Ismail N, Collins P, Rogers S, at al. Drug survival of fumaric acid esters for psoriasis: a retrospective study. Br J Dermatol 2014; 17:1397–1402.

Mrowietz U, Christophers E, Altmeyer P. Treatment of psoriasis with fumaric acid esters: results of a prospective multicentre study. German Multicentre Study. Br J Dermatol 1998; 138:456–460.

Nast A, Boehncke WH, Mrowietz U, et al. S3 - Guidelines on the treatment of psoriasis vulgaris (English version). Update. J Dtsch Dermatol Ges 2012; 10 (suppl 2):S1–S95.

Rostami Yazdi M, Mrowietz U. Fumaric acid esters. Clin Dermatol 2008; 26: 522–526.

Van Oosten BW, Killestein J, Barkhof F, et al. PML in a patient treated with dimethyl fumarate from a compounding pharmacy. N Engl J Med 2013; 368:1658–1659.

Glucocorticoids

Dermatologic indications

- Flares of atopic dermatitis, pemphigus vulgaris, bullous pemphigoid, systemic lupus erythematosus, pyoderma gangrenosum, many other inflammatory dermatoses

- *Also used for:* eosinophilic fasciitis, pruritic urticarial papules and plaques of pregnancy (PUPPP), pemphigoid gestationis, relapsing polychondritis, dermatomyositis, polymorphic light eruption, morphea, calciphylaxis, linear IgA bullous dermatosis, aphthous stomatitis, epidermolysis bullosa aquisita, acute graft versus host disease, granulomatous cheilitis, Hailey-Hailey disease, Kawasaki disease, necrobiosis lipodica, acne fulminans, urticaria (acute/severe), Langerhans cell histiocytosis (with vinblastine in children)

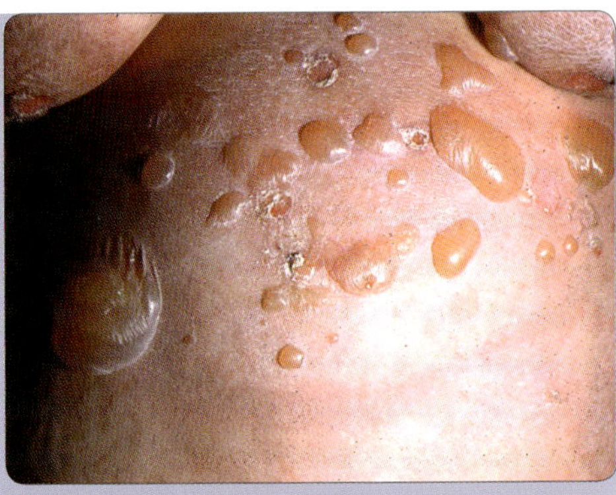

Figure 42.1 Bullous pemphigoid. Tense bullae on urticated, erythematous abdominal skin of an elderly woman.

Background

Glucocorticoids are an effective therapeutic option for many inflammatory skin diseases.

Glucocorticoids ('steroids') are steroid hormones, produced in the adrenal glands, the production of which is controlled by the hypothalamic-pituitary-adrenal (HPA) axis. Steroids act through binding to the intracellular glucocorticoid receptor, which induces gene transcription; they are potently anti-inflammatory and immunosuppressive. They also have metabolic effects, regulating glucose, protein, lipid, and calcium levels.

Cortisol is the main endogenous glucocorticoid found in humans. Synthetic glucocorticoids have been developed, either as replacement therapy in patients with cortisol deficiency or as immunosuppressant therapy. These vary in their potency compared to cortisol (**Table 42.1**).

The most commonly prescribed synthetic glucocorticoid in the UK is prednisolone. In the US, the inactive precursor prednisone is commonly prescribed; this is converted to prednisolone by hepatic metabolism.

Dermatologic prescribing

- Widely used for acute flares of inflammatory dermatoses or as an adjunct to initiating systemic immunosuppressant therapy for chronic diseases

- Glucocorticoids should be taken once daily, preferably in the morning

Table 42.1 Synthetic glucocorticoids and their equivalent dosages

Glucocorticoid	Equivalent dose
Prednisolone	5 mg
Betamethasone	750 µg
Dexamethasone	750 µg
Methylprednisolone	4 mg
Triamcinolone	4 mg
Prednisone	5 mg
Hydrocortisone (cortisol)	20 mg

- For severe disease, an intravenous route may be preferable to oral therapy, both for effective absorption and rapid onset of action

- Both prednisolone and prednisone are commonly prescribed at doses of 0.5–1 mg/kg, although higher doses (up to 2 mg/kg) are occasionally used

- It is critical to regularly review glucocorticoid doses to maximize efficacy while minimizing side effects

Cautions

- *Adrenal suppression:* prolonged therapy with steroids leads to adrenal atrophy through HPA axis suppression, which can persist for years after treatment cessation. Rapid withdrawal of exogenous glucocorticoids can precipitate acute adrenal insufficiency, which can result in death. Inter-current illness, surgery, or trauma in a patient receiving glucocorticoid therapy will require an increased steroid dose to compensate for a diminished adrenocortical response to these physiologic stressors

- *Steroid treatment withdrawal:* gradual withdrawal of systemic treatment is imperative in those patients who have:

  - \>3 weeks of treatment at any dose
  - Taken ≥40 mg of prednisolone or prednisone daily for longer than 1 week
  - Had several repeated courses within a few months
  - Taken repeated doses in the evening
  - An additional course of steroids (short or long) within 1 year of stopping long-term therapy

- *Infections:* increased susceptibility to infections, especially varicella (chickenpox) and measles. Infections may present late and in an atypical fashion

- *Metabolic:* elevated blood glucose levels; diabetic patients may require altered doses of their diabetic medication

- *Hepatic derangement:* plasma concentrations of glucocorticoids may be increased

- *Children:* growth restriction possible (may be irreversible)

- *Pregnancy:* prolonged or repeated courses may lead to intrauterine growth restriction

Common problems

- *Osteoporosis:* initiation of calcium and vitamin D supplements, bisphosphonate therapy, and a baseline bone density scan is recommended when commencing prolonged therapy, especially in those over 65 years of age

- *Skin:* ecchymoses, skin atrophy, bruising, petechiae, poor healing, facial erythema, hirsutism

- *Psychiatric:* can induce insomnia, nightmares, euphoria, suicidal thoughts, and psychosis.

Caution needed in patients with psychiatric disorders

- *Endocrine:* diabetes can be worsened or precipitated. Cushing's syndrome (moon facies, striae, acne) may occur

- *Gastrointestinal:* dyspepsia, pancreatitis, esophageal ulcers, and candidiasis

- *Miscellaneous:* weight gain, sodium and water retention, hypertension, muscle weakness, avascular necrosis, and cataracts are all recognized side effects

Further reading

Dixon WG, Bansback N. Understanding the side effects of glucocorticoid therapy: shining a light on a drug everyone thinks they know. Ann Rheum Dis 2012; 71:1761–1764.

Hoes JN, Jacobs JWD, Bijlsma JWJ. Glucocorticoids are forever? Rheumatology 2011; 50:1940.

Treatment pearls

- Even a daily dose of 7.5 mg of prednisolone or prednisone is enough to suppress the HPA axis

- Topical steroids may rarely cause HPA suppression; topical use of a 50 g tube of clobetasol propionate 0.05% cream in 1 week is equivalent to 7.5 mg of prednisolone daily

- Early morning doses are better tolerated

- Patients should be given a steroid card to carry

- Do not prescribe prednisone in patients with pre-existing hepatic disease as it will not be converted into physiologically active prednisolone

- Psoriasis can be exacerbated on withdrawal of glucocorticoid treatment

Hydroxyurea (hydroxycarbamide)

Dermatologic indications

- Psoriasis
- *Also used for:* hypereosinophilic syndrome

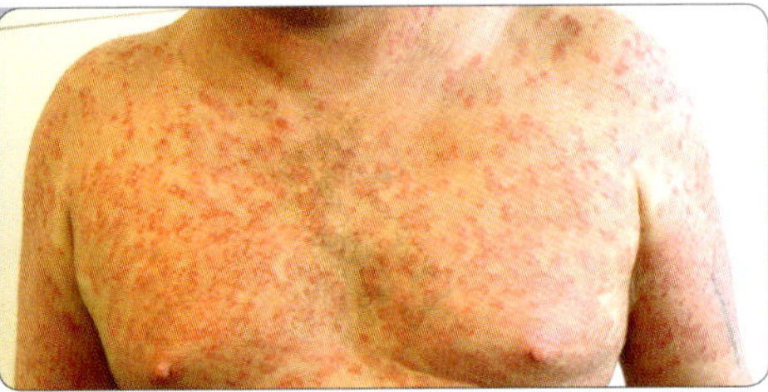

Figure 43.1 Widespread plaques of psoriasis on the chest and arms of a middle-aged man.

Background

Hydroxyurea inhibits DNA synthesis in replicating cells by inhibiting ribonucleotide reductase and bringing about S-phase cell cycle arrest.

All individuals taking hydroxycarbamide develop macrocytosis, which rarely leads to anemia.

Psoriasis

- Hydroxycarbamide has been used off-license for the treatment of psoriasis since 1970
- The use of hydroxycarbamide for psoriasis has been largely superseded by the introduction of immunomodulatory drugs and biologic agents
- In patients in whom standard treatments are contraindicated or ineffective, hydroxycarbamide may still have a role

Hypereosinophilic syndrome

- A group of disorders characterized by a persistent eosinophilia with eosinophil-induced tissue inflammation resulting in organ dysfunction or damage
- Cutaneous features are variable in hypereosinophilic syndrome, but can include urticarial, edematous, papular, or nodular lesions
- Hydroxycarbamide is used as a second line agent in the management of this condition

Dermatologic prescribing

- *Dose:* 0.5–2.0 g per day
- Gradual dose escalation depending on the patient's response may allow for safer monitoring of side effects
- *Monitoring:* complete blood count and renal and liver function tests are recommended weekly for four weeks at induction and dose increments, thereafter extending to every 4–12 weeks once the dose is stable

Cautions

- Pregnancy and breast feeding:
- Hydroxycarbamide is contraindicated
- Men should use contraception during therapy and for at least 3 months after completion
- The risk to fetal development is likely to be low, but contraception for women of child-bearing age is advised

- Bone marrow suppression: leukopenia (leukocytes $<2.5 \times 10^9$/L), thrombocytopenia (platelets $<100 \times 10^9$/L), or severe anemia

Common problems

Gastrointestinal

- Bowel disturbance including diarrhea or constipation are commonly reported

Hematologic

- Bone marrow suppression occurs 7–10 days after commencing treatment
- Mild leukopenia is common, but profound suppression is less frequent
- Treatment should be discontinued or withheld in the event of leukopenia (leukocytes $<2.5 \times 10^9$/L), thrombocytopenia (platelets $<100 \times 10^9$/L), or severe anemia, until levels have risen significantly
- Myelosuppression resolves on discontinuation of treatment
- Macrocytosis due to megaloblastosis is extremely common and unresponsive to replacement with vitamin B12 or folic acid

Cutaneous

- The proportion of patients that experience mucocutaneous side effects varies widely between studies (6.6–65.5%)
- Dry skin and occasionally pruritus may be seen
- Pigmentation of the nails, skin, and mucosal surfaces is commonly reported
- Rarely, leg ulceration requiring discontinuation of treatment may occur in patients on hydroxycarbamide (more common in patients treated for hematologic disease). In addition, nail dystrophy and dermatomyositis-like cutaneous eruptions are reported
- Patients on long-term treatment should be advised to avoid excessive sun exposure (levels leading to tanning or burning) due to the potential increased risk of skin malignancy

Further reading

Belgi G, Friedmann PS. Traditional therapies: glucocorticoids, azathioprine, methotrexate, hydroxyurea. Clin Exp Derm 2002; 27:546–554.

Griffiths CEM, Clark CM, Chalmers RJG, et al. A systematic review of treatments for severe psoriasis. Health Technol Assess 2000; 4:1–125.

Kumar B, Saraswat A, Kaur I. Mucocutaneous adverse effects of hydroxyurea: a prospective study of 30 psoriasis patients. Clin Exp Derm 2002; 27:8–13.

Treatment pearls

- Hydroxycarbamide is ineffective in the treatment of psoriatic arthritis
- Erythrodermic psoriasis may respond to treatment with hydroxycarbamide
- Generalized pustular psoriasis has been successfully managed with hydroxycarbamide in a small number of cases
- Hydroxycarbamide can be used with caution in combination with other systemic therapies (e.g. cyclosporine, methotrexate, and acitretin), however, with the advent of biologic therapy, this is rarely necessary
- Patients should be informed to expect a delay in improvement of psoriasis of 4–8 weeks while the treatment reaches its maximal effect
- Topical treatments for psoriasis should be used in addition to hydroxycarbamide in order to optimize disease control and reduce the dose and/or need for additional systemic therapy
- Macrocytosis can act as a reliable biologic readout of concordance with treatment. Care should be taken when the mean corpuscular volume exceeds 105 fL as anemia is more likely
- Lower doses should be used in the elderly as they are more likely to be sensitive to the effects of hydroxycarbamide
- Evidence exists for the use of hydroxycarbamide in the management of HIV via the inhibition of HIV DNA synthesis and HIV replication
- Theoretically, hydroxycarbamide may therefore be a therapeutic option when managing patients with both HIV and psoriasis. However, no studies have been conducted to support this
- Care should be taken on discontinuation of treatment due to the potential risk of rebound of the patient's psoriasis

Intravenous immunoglobulin

Dermatologic indications

- Dermatomyositis, pemphigus vulgaris, pemphigus foliaceus, scleromyxedema, Stevens–Johnson syndrome
- *Also used for:* toxic epidermal necrolysis, bullous pemphigoid, cicatricial pemphigoid, epidermolysis bullosa acquisita, linear IgA disease, pemphigoid gestationis, pyoderma gangrenosum, atopic dermatitis (atopic eczema)

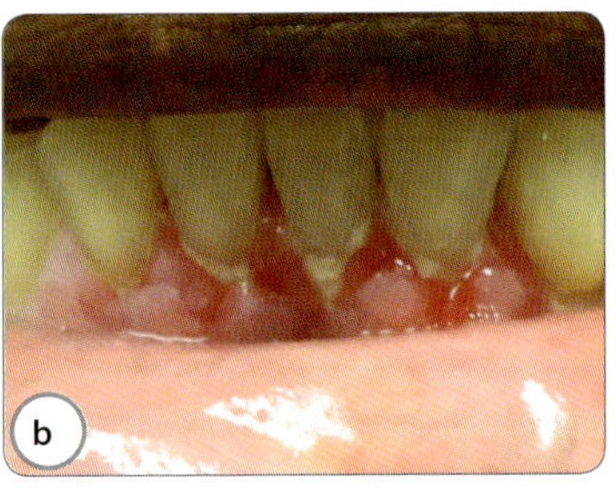

Background

Intravenous immunoglobulin contains polyvalent IgG antibodies fractionated and purified from plasma pooled from 3,000 to 10,000 screened human donors.

The type and concentration of other components (e.g. IgA, sugar, salt, protein) vary according to the specific product.

Anti-inflammatory and immunomodulatory mechanisms are poorly understood, but are believed to be mediated largely through the constant (Fc) region of IgG. The Fc region may bind to Fc receptors on phagocytes, preventing activation by pathogenic antigens; to neonatal Fc receptors on endothelial cells, leading to the clearance of unbound antibodies including autoantibodies; or to complement components, inhibiting formation of the membrane attack complex.

Dermatologic prescribing

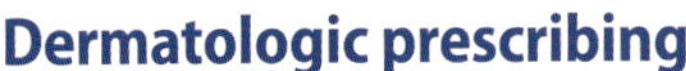

- *Most dermatologic indications:* high-dose monthly regimen. Total dose each month is 2 g/kg of ideal or adjusted body weight, divided evenly over 2–5 consecutive days (e.g. 1 g/kg/day for 2 consecutive days) administered every 4 weeks
- *Stevens–Johnson syndrome and toxic epidermal necrolysis:* 1 g/kg/day for 3 days consecutively (total dose 3 g/kg), ideally administered within 48 hours of disease onset
- *Route:* intravenous (most common), subcutaneous (SCIg) is also available
- Often used as an adjuvant to systemic corticosteroids and/or other immunosuppressive agents

Cautions

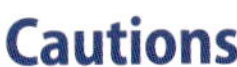

- *Thrombosis:* risk factors include hypercoagulable conditions (including malignancy), indwelling catheters, and prior thrombosis. Only rarely reported in the absence of risk factors

Figure 44.1 (a) Violaceous erythema and poikiloderma on the photoexposed neck ('V-neck sign') and upper chest in a patient with dermatomyositis. (b) Desquamative gingivitis in a patient with pemphigus vulgaris.

- *Acute kidney injury:* risk is lower with sucrose-free products; if occurs, it is generally reversible
- *Anaphylaxis:* extremely rare but possible in IgA-deficient patients
- *Blood-borne pathogen transmission:* has not yet been reported with IVIG made by current standards; may consider monitoring for HIV and hepatitis B and C given theoretical risk
- *Medication interactions:* nephrotoxic medications may increase the risk of acute kidney injury. Estrogen derivatives may increase the risk of thrombosis. MMR and varicella virus vaccines may be less effective if IVIG is given within 2 weeks and 2 months of vaccination, respectively, or if the vaccines are given within 6 months of IVIG use
- *Pregnancy/lactation risk:* Risk in pregnancy has not been ruled out, and risks must be carefully weighed up against potential benefits. Safety during breastfeeding is unknown, although limited data, primarily in post-partum patients with multiple sclerosis treated with doses of IVIG lower than those typically used for dermatologic indications, suggests that IVIG may be well-

tolerated by both mother and infant during breastfeeding

Common problems

- IVIG is generally well-tolerated, and the side effect profile is considered minimal

- Tension headache, which may be severe, is the most common side effect. Adequate pre-infusion hydration and slowing the rate of infusion ameliorate the risk; severe headache may be treated with an intravenous saline infusion. Prescribing intravenous hydration concomitantly with future infusions may prevent additional headaches

- Self-limited aseptic meningitis may develop within 2 days of an infusion; history of migraine may be risk factor

- Infusion reactions:

- Include fever, chills, malaise, flushing, gastrointestinal upset, and/or musculoskeletal pain

- Rare reactions with dyspnea, tachypnea, chest pain, and/or urticaria may be differentiated from anaphylaxis by delayed onset during an infusion and lack of associated hypotension

- Tend to be self-limited and lessen with continued use of an IVIG product

- Thrombosis is rare, but caution should be used in the setting of malignancy or other hypercoagulable risk factors. Consultation with a hematologist may be warranted to weigh risks versus benefits in such cases

Further reading

Çakmak SK, Çakmak A, Gönül M, Kiliç A, Gül Ü. Intravenous immunoglobulin therapy in dermatology: an update. Inflamm Allergy Drug Targets 2013; 12:132–146.

Enk A; European Dermatology Forum Guideline Subcommittee. Guidelines on the use of high-dose intravenous immunoglobulin in dermatology. Eur J Dermatol 2009; 19:90–98.

Prins C, Gelfand EW, French LE. Intravenous immunoglobulin: properties, mode of action and practical use in dermatology. Acta Derm Venereol 2007; 87:206–218.

Smith DI, Swamy PM, Heffernan MP. Off-label uses of biologics in dermatology: interferon and intravenous immunoglobulin (part 1 of 2). J Am Acad Dermatol. 2007; 56:e1–e54.

Treatment pearls

- Selection of the formulation of IVIG is often based upon availability and patient comorbidities:

- *No comorbidities:* consider Gamunex-C and other sucrose-free, low-IgA products

- *Kidney disease:* avoid Carimune NF (contains sucrose)

- *Thrombosis risk:* consider Gammaked and Gamunex-C (lowest osmolarity), and consider limiting dose to 500 mg/kg/day

- *IgA deficiency:* consider Gammagard S/D (IgA <1 μg/mL in a 5% solution) or Flebogamma DIF (lowest in IgA)

- *Fluid overload risk:* consider Gammagard liquid (lacks added sodium or albumin)

- Intravenous administration is usually preferred for dermatologic indications as subcutaneous administration often requires multiple injections to achieve an adequate dose

- IVIG is often used in combination with rituximab for bullous diseases

- Side effects of IVIG may be prevented or minimized by:

- Intravenous hydration prior to or concurrently with an infusion

- Dividing the total monthly dose over a greater number of consecutive days

- Slowing the infusion rate

- Delivering by subcutaneous route

- Given the risk of thrombosis, patients should be advised to avoid prolonged immobilization such as air travel after an infusion

- In most dermatologic diseases, IVIG is not thought to induce remission, and prolonged courses of therapy are often required

- As patients improve, the interval between infusions may be increased gradually from 4 weeks to 5 weeks and so forth, with some patients able to tolerate infusions spaced at 7–10 week intervals

Isotretinoin

Dermatologic indications

- *Acne and variants:* severe recalcitrant nodular acne, acne fulminans
- *Also used for:* hidradenitis suppurativa, severe papulopustular rosacea
- *Occasionally used for:* cutaneous T-cell lymphoma, squamous cell skin cancers, xeroderma pigmentosum, ichthyoses (harlequin and lamellar types), Darier's disease, cutaneous lupus erythematosus, lichen planus

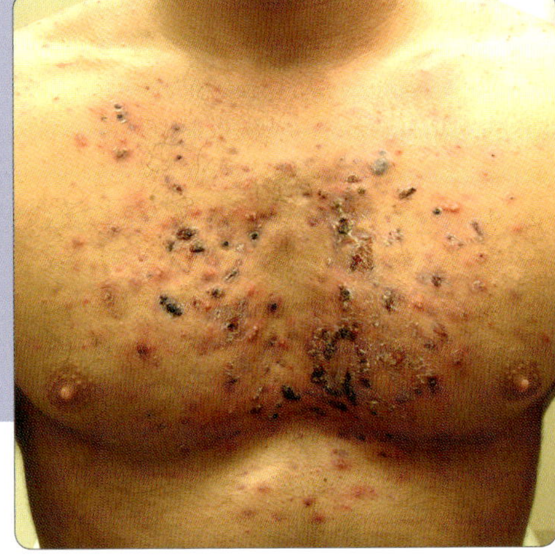

Figure 45.1 Acne vulgaris. Severe inflammatory papules, pustules, and nodules on the chest of an adult male. Note the presence of several deep scars corresponding to prior acne lesions. The patient was successfully treated with a course of isotretinoin.

Background

Isotretinoin acts as a pro-drug; downstream metabolites bind to retinoic acid receptors (RARs) and retinoid X receptors (RXRs) and regulate gene transcription.

It induces apoptosis in sebaceous gland cells, reducing sebum production, and decreases hyperkeratinization, thus reducing comedone formation.

It exerts an antimicrobial effect on *Propionibacterium acnes* bacterium.

Its mechanism of action explains its benefit in acne as well as in a variety of other dermatologic conditions that affect the pilo-sebaceous unit.

Dermatologic prescribing

- *Route:* oral
- *Oral dosing:* 0.5–1 mg/kg/day for 15–20 weeks. Goal cumulative dose: 120–150 mg/kg. Adults with severe scarring or cysts primarily involving the trunk may require up to 2 mg/kg/day. A second course of therapy may be initiated after >2 months off therapy for relapse. Moderate acne (adults and children 12–17 years of age): 20 mg/day for 6 months. Can be taken as single or divided doses
- May discontinue treatment earlier if total lesion count decreases by 70%; may see a higher risk of recurrence in patients who do not receive the full course of therapy
- Administration with meals, particularly if high in fat, enhances absorption
- Pre-treatment investigations include complete blood count, liver function tests, lipid panel. Repeat monthly (less frequent monitoring in some countries)
- All women of child-bearing potential require a negative pregnancy screen before initiation of isotretinoin, monthly during treatment, and one month following completion of therapy. In some countries such as the UK, women at no risk of pregnancy may opt out of the pregnancy prevention program if the prescribing physician agrees, and if they sign a second consent form stating that they are at no risk of pregnancy. A pre-start negative pregnancy test is still advised
- Two forms of contraception (usually one hormonal, one barrier) are recommended for females from 1 month before therapy, during therapy, and 1 month after therapy. Oral contraceptive pills containing only progesterone are not recommended alone

Cautions

- Contraindicated in hepatic failure, cautioned in hepatic impairment, renal disease or diabetes
- *Interactions:* isotretinoin should not be used in conjunction with tetracyclines due to a risk of benign intracranial hypertension. Patients should avoid additional vitamin A supplementation, especially through multivitamins
- *Allergy:* allergy to peanut or soy is listed as a contraindication in preparations containing arachis oil. However, recent studies suggest that anaphylactic reactions to isotretinoin in such patients are very unlikely. As a minimum, the first isotretinoin dose should be given in an environment with full resuscitation facilities in patients with peanut or soy allergy
- *Liver:* patients should limit alcohol consumption while on isotretinoin

- *Gastrointestinal:* although some controversy exists linking isotretinoin to inflammatory bowel disease (IBD), recent meta-analyses do not support this claim
- *Musculoskeletal:* premature epiphyseal plate closure may rarely occur in patients who have not yet met their growth potential
- *Teratogenicity:* isotretinoin exposure in utero, even only for a few days, is associated with a high risk for malformations. Pregnancy screening is required for all women of child-bearing potential prior to commencement of treatment, throughout the course, and for 1 month after discontinuation
- *Psychiatric:* the precise risk of mood disturbance with isotretinoin remains unclear, but is considered low. However, depression, mania, psychosis, and aggressive/violent behavior have been noted in some patients taking isotretinoin. There is an established association between acne and depression. Mood should be evaluated in every patient prior to starting isotretinoin. A useful set of screening questions would include:

For most of the last 2 weeks, have you:

- Been feeling unusually sad or fed up?
- Lost interest in things that used to interest you, or gave you pleasure?
- Been significantly more agitated, irritable or short-tempered?

- *Other:* May cause hearing loss and tinnitus. Medication should be discontinued at first sign of either

Common problems

- *Expected:* cheilitis, xerosis, intermittent epistaxis, arthralgias, myalgias, and back pain
- *Frequent:* photosensitivity, alopecia, impetigo (*Staphylococcus aureus*), acne flares upon treatment initiation
- *Lipids:* increased lipids (most commonly triglycerides) in 25% of patients
- *Hepatobiliary:* increased transaminases
- *Hematologic:* anemia, thrombocytopenia, neutropenia
- *Ocular:* xerophthalmia, worsened night vision, conjunctivitis, blepharitis
- *Management of adverse effects:* dose reduction is usually effective

Further reading

Amichai B, Shemer A, Grunwald MH. Low-dose isotretinoin in the treatment of acne vulgaris. J Am Acad Dermatol 2006; 54:644–646.

Cyrulnik AA, Viola KV, Gewirtzman AJ, Cohen SR. High-dose isotretinoin in acne vulgaris: improved treatment outcomes and quality of life. Int J Dermatol 2012; 51:1123–1130.

Layton A. The use of isotretinoin in acne. Dermatoendocrinol 2009; 1:162–169.

Treatment pearls

- Therapy is ideally stopped when patients have had at least 2 weeks without further new acne lesions
- Acne may initially worsen with isotretinoin therapy; however, this flare will typically subside with continued treatment
- For severe acne or acne fulminans, oral glucocorticoids (0.5–1.0 mg/kg/day) may be administered before or during the initial 2–4 weeks of isotretinoin therapy to decrease severity of the acne flare
- Oral isotretinoin is best absorbed when taken with a fatty meal due to its lipophilicity
- The severity of cheilitis (dry lips) acts as a biomarker for dose effect
- Prescribing of isotretinoin occurs through the pharmacy regulatory program iPLEDGE in the US, and the Pregnancy Prevention Programme in Europe
- Negative side effects are usually dose dependent, but lower doses may require an extended treatment course to achieve the target dose
- Pilots should not take isotretinoin (risk of loss of night vision)
- Isotretinoin should not be withheld due to concern for causing IBD, but consideration of alternatives in individuals with a strong family history of IBD may be warranted
- Patients should not donate blood during treatment or for one month after completing treatment to avoid possible exposure of isotretinoin-containing blood products to women of childbearing age
- Isotretinoin can interfere with wound healing, therefore, surgery and cosmetic procedures are best avoided during treatment
- Cosmetic interventions to manage scarring from acne should be deferred until at least 6 months after isotretinoin

Methotrexate

Dermatologic indications

- Psoriasis
- Cutaneous lupus, dermatomyositis, morphea , sarcoidosis and other granulomatous dermatitides
- *Also used for:* atopic dermatitis, alopecia areata, lichen planus, bullous pemphigoid, pemphigus vulgaris, CD30+ cutaneous lymphoproliferative disorders

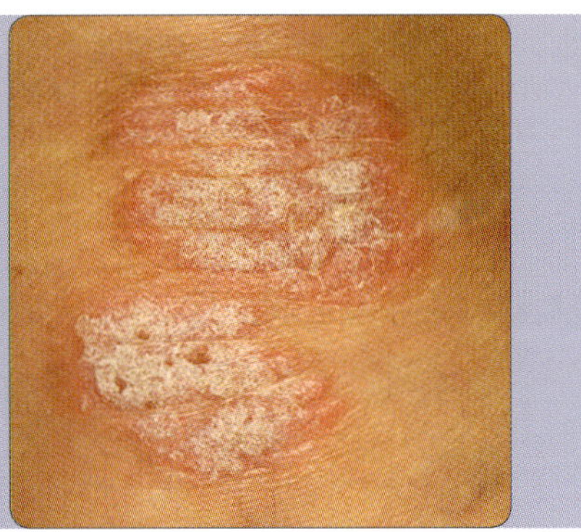

Figure 46.1 Plaque psoriasis. Well-demarcated erythematous plaques with silvery scale.

Background

Methotrexate is an antimetabolite that inhibits dihydrofolate reductase, depleting intracellular folate. Co-administration of folic acid may reduce many side effects.

Methotrexate inhibits lymphocyte proliferation by increasing production of adenosine deaminase, a potent anti-inflammatory protein. Adenosine has many anti-inflammatory effects, including reduction of lymphocyte migration into tissues and cytokine secretion. This effect is thought to explain methotrexate's anti-inflammatory benefit in a wide variety of dermatologic disorders.

Dermatologic prescribing

- For dermatologic purposes, methotrexate is prescribed in a low-dose weekly regimen. The maximum dose is 25–30 mg/week. Patients are often started on 10 mg/week for 1–2 weeks prior to escalation to full dose
- Methotrexate can be taken orally, or injected subcutaneously or intramuscularly. The IV formulation is rarely used in dermatology
- Oral methotrexate is dispensed as 2.5 mg tablets. The total dose may be taken all at once or taken in two doses 12 hours apart (i.e. 10 mg/week = 4 × 2.5 mg tablets once weekly, or 2 × 2.5 mg tablets every 12 hours for 24 hours, once weekly)
- Injectable methotrexate is formulated as 25 mg/mL. It is also available in 7.5 mg to 30 mg doses (2.5 mg increments) as a pen injection. Injections are once weekly
- Folic acid is prescribed with methotrexate, generally as 1 mg daily or 5 mg weekly
- Regular monitoring of complete blood counts and renal and liver function is essential. A typical monitoring schedule is checking these at baseline, 2 weeks, 6 weeks, and every 2–3 months thereafter

Cautions

- *Liver disease:* hepatitis B or C, advanced stage fatty liver, excessive alcohol intake, other causes of hepatic impairment
- *Renal disease:* methotrexate has predominantly renal excretion; the dose is reduced for creatinine clearance <30 mL/min. It is contraindicated with creatinine clearance <10 mL/min
- *Medication interactions:* methotrexate has multiple drug interactions; potential interactions should be assessed in all patients. Tetracyclines, trimethoprim, sulfonamides, and NSAIDs are common drugs that interact with methotrexate. Short courses in young, healthy patients with normal renal function are unlikely to be problematic, but co-administration in elderly patients with reduced GFR should be especially restricted
- *Pregnancy/lactation risk:* contraindicated in pregnancy and lactation, and in both men and women trying to conceive; discontinue 3 months prior to conception
- *Immunosuppression:* HIV, bone marrow suppression

Common problems

- *Gastrointestinal upset:* most often the day following oral methotrexate
- *Stomatitis:* may occur but is less common at lower doses and with folic acid administration
- *Bone marrow suppression:* generally manifests with mild leukopenia or anemia, and usually does not require treatment discontinuation. Increased doses of folic acid can improve mild changes, whereas folinic acid (leucovorin)

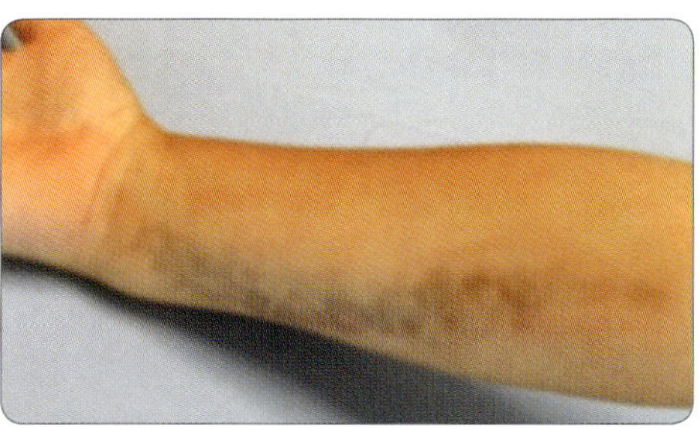

Figure 46.2 Linear morphea. Linear indurated, hyperpigmented plaque with subtle erythema.

may be administered to reverse bone marrow suppression

- *Hepatotoxicity:* mild transaminitis (ALT <2–3 times the upper limit of normal) generally does not reflect serious underlying pathology, and is managed with dose adjustments. Chronic hepatotoxicity is less common than previously thought. Hepatic panels are monitored regularly; further testing is directed towards abnormal findings. In the US and UK, routine liver biopsies are no longer performed. Ultrasonography and/or transient elastography is often used in patients on methotrexate with liver function test abnormalities. Current evidence does not support the use of procollagen 3 *N*-terminal peptide (P3NP) in isolation to monitor for liver fibrosis. Liver fibrosis may be more common in patients with obesity, diabetes, fatty liver, or those who consume alcohol. Alcohol intake should be limited in all patients

Further reading

Bangert CA, Costner MI. Methotrexate in dermatology. Dermatol Ther 2007; 20:216–228.

Chakravarty K, Mc Donald H, Pullar T, et al. BSR/BHPR guideline for disease-modifying anti-rheumatic drug (DMARD) therapy in consultation with the British Association of Dermatologists. Rheumatology 2008; 47:924–925.

Kalb RE, Strober B, Weinstein G, Lebwohl M. Methotrexate and psoriasis: 2009 National Psoriasis Foundation Consensus Conference. J Am Acad Dermatol 2009; 60:824–837.

Treatment pearls

- GI is the most common side effect with oral methotrexate, and can be managed by:
  - Increasing the folic acid dose up to 5 mg daily; this approach is first-line in many centers
  - Dividing the methotrexate dose into two doses administered evenly over 24 hours
  - Adding an anti-nausea medication such as ondansetron before and after the dose of methotrexate
  - Adding folinic acid (typically 10–25 mg, matched to the dose of methotrexate, e.g. 20 mg folinic acid for a patient on 20 mg of methotrexate) 12 hours following the dose of methotrexate
  - Switching from the oral to the injectable formulation of methotrexate; this is likely the most effective way to eliminate gastrointestinal side effects from oral methotrexate
- Patients with psoriasis generally require lower doses of methotrexate than patients with autoimmune connective tissue diseases or granulomatous conditions
- At higher dermatologic doses (20–30 mg/week), switching from oral to injectable methotrexate may improve systemic absorption and thus efficacy
- Some centers avoid folic acid on the same day as methotrexate, while others give it daily
- Patients are often concerned about the risk of hair loss with methotrexate, but with dermatologic doses, scalp involvement by the underlying condition (e.g. cutaneous lupus or dermatomyositis) is more likely to be the cause. In these cases, the hair loss is likely to improve with methotrexate
- Narrowband UVB phototherapy can be combined with methotrexate for patients with psoriasis
- In general, patients should continue to use topical treatment when starting methotrexate
- Methotrexate generally reaches maximal efficacy after 3 months, and patients should be counseled regarding this time-frame. Three months is considered an appropriate trial of methotrexate when given at an adequate dose
- Monitoring creatinine clearance is especially important in the elderly and in those with multiple co-morbidities given that fluctuations in renal function can substantially alter methotrexate levels

Mycophenolate mofetil

Dermatologic indications

- Immunobullous diseases: pemphigus vulgaris, bullous pemphigoid, epidermolysis bullosa acquisita, cicatricial pemphigoid
- Chronic eczema and atopic dermatitis
- *Also used for:* cutaneous lupus erythematosus, dermatomyositis, cutaneous vasculitis, pyoderma gangrenosum and other neutrophilic dermatoses, cutaneous Crohn disease, sarcoidosis, lichen planopilaris, chronic urticaria, cutaneous sclerosis in systemic sclerosis (scleroderma), morphea, and eosinophilic fasciitis

Background

Mycophenolate mofetil (MMF) is a prodrug that is converted to mycophenolic acid (MPA), which inhibits inosine monophosphate dehydrogenase and thereby purine synthesis.

It suppresses T-cell mediated function and reduces antibody production by B-cells.

It reduces the recruitment of inflammatory cells by altering the expression of cell surface adhesion molecules.

Dermatologic prescribing

- Dosage forms: 250 mg tablet or capsule, 500 mg tablet or capsule, oral suspension 200 mg/mL, or powder for intravenous injection
- Initial dosing in adults is typically 500 mg twice daily. The dose can be titrated up to 1500 mg twice daily
- Mycophenolate mofetil is available as a generic drug. The original branded version is called Cellcept
- An alternative product is Myofortic, which is mycophenolic acid as mycophenolate sodium. This drug produces similar effects to mycophenolate mofetil, but the dosing is not equivalent. 720 mg of mycophenolic acid is equivalent to 1 g of mycophenolate mofetil
- Although there are no specific guidelines for monitoring early in therapy, measurements of complete blood counts and transaminases are typically performed at baseline, 2 and 6 weeks after initiation of therapy, and then every 3 months thereafter

Cautions

Hematologic

- Cytopenias are possible and are dose-related

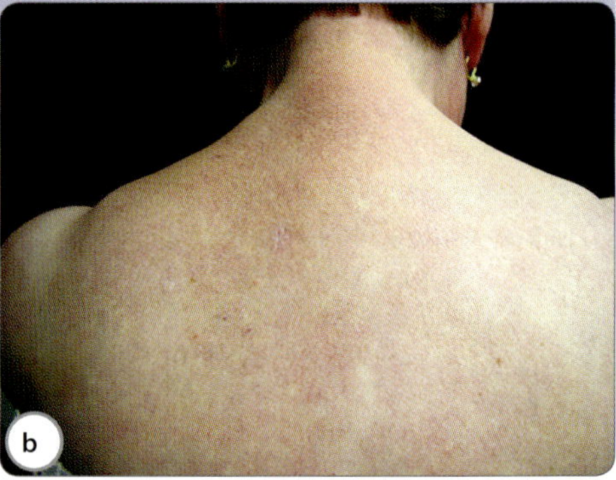

Figure 47.1 Dermatomyositis (a) before and (b) after mycophenolate mofetil.

Malignancy

- There is a potential risk of post-transplantation lymphoproliferative disease or lymphoma
- There is an increased risk of non-melanoma skin cancer, particularly squamous cell carcinoma. However, this risk is lower for mycophenolate mofetil than for azathioprine

Idiosyncratic reactions

- None are known

Infectious complications

- Infections including viral, bacterial, atypical mycobacterial, and fungal
- Progressive multifocal leukoencephalopathy (rare)

Medication interactions

- Drugs that may decrease the level of mycophenolic acid through an effect on absorption include antacids, proton pump inhibitors, and iron containing compounds
- Drugs that may decrease the level of mycophenolic acid through impairment of enterohepatic circulation include antibiotics and bile acid sequestrants

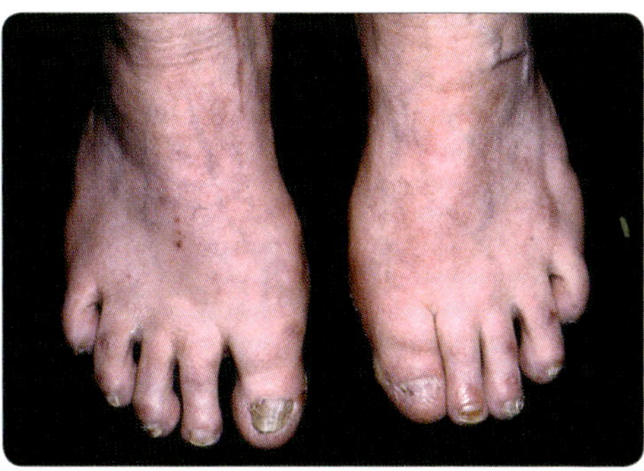

Figure 47.2 Epidermolysis bullosa acquisita treated with mycophenolate mofetil. Chronic skin fragility is most apparent on the digits. Subsequent scarring and loss of several nail plates can be seen.

- Live vaccines are contraindicated due to risk of infection and potential decrease in efficacy
- Mycophenolate mofetil might increase levels of the following agents: antiviral agents, bronchodilators including theophylline, phenytoin, and cyclosporine

Pregnancy/lactation risk

- Mycophenolate mofetil is contraindicated in pregnancy; its use is associated with first term pregnancy loss and fetal malformations
- A program for safety in pregnancy known as Mycophenolate REMS (Risk Evaluation and Mitigation Strategy) has been devised and is mandated by the Food and Drug Administration in the US
- Mycophenolate might be associated with decreased lactation and with immune suppression in neonates who are breast fed

Immunosuppression

- Concomitant use of other immunosuppressive therapy with mycophenolate mofetil increases the risk of infection and level of immune suppression

Treatment pearls

- The onset of action for mycophenolate mofetil in dermatologic disease is roughly 12 weeks at 'full' dose. Cessation prior to that time is an inadequate trial
- Although an increased risk of non-melanoma skin cancer is linked to mycophenolate mofetil in allograft recipients, this association is not as well established in dermatologic disease
- Following control of disease, gradual reduction and possible cessation of therapy is possible, but should be done slowly
- For patients with pemphigus vulgaris, the monitoring of anti-desmoglein antibody titers may help to direct when it is safe to reduce the dose

Common problems

- Nausea, diarrhea, vomiting, anorexia
- Urinary urgency, dysuria, sterile pyuria

Further reading

Edge JC, Outland JD, Dempsey JR, Callen JP. Mycophenolate mofetil as an effective corticosteroid-sparing therapy for recalcitrant dermatomyositis. Arch Dermatol 2006; 142:65–69.

Eskin-Schwartz M, David M, Mimouni D. Mycophenolate mofetil for the management of autoimmune bullous diseases. Immunol Allergy Clin North Am 2012; 32:309–315;

George L, Hamann I, Chen K, et al. An analysis of the dermatological uses of mycophenolate mofetil in a tertiary hospital. J Dermatolog Treat 2015; 26:63–66.

Schadt CR, Zwerner JP. Mycophenolate mofetil and mycophenolic acid. In: Wolverton SE (Ed). Comprehensive Dermatologic Therapy, 3rd Edn. Philadelphia: Elsevier-Saunders, 2012. pp.190–198.

Dermatologic indications

- Erythema nodosum leprosum (ENL), actinic prurigo, aphthous stomatitis, cutaneous lupus erythematosus, recurrent erythema multiforme, Kaposi sarcoma, nodular prurigo, chronic graft versus host disease, and Behçet's disease

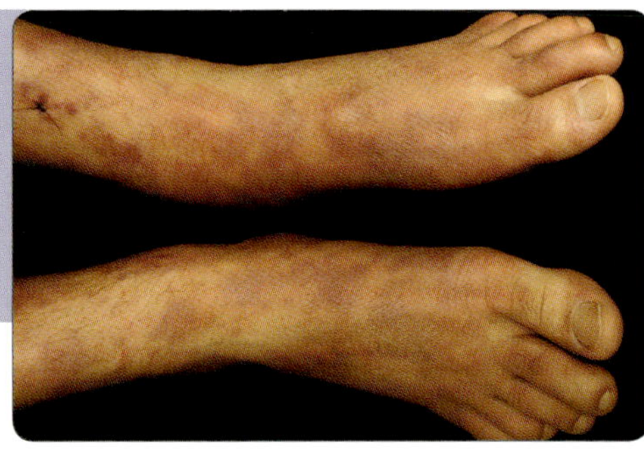

Figure 48.1 A young Brazilian man with erythema nodosum leprosum; he was treated with systemic glucocorticoids and thalidomide.

Background

Thalidomide was originally licensed as an antiemetic during pregnancy but was identified as the cause of an epidemic of severe birth defects during the 1950s. Due to this significant side effect, its use was banned and its license revoked.

However, thalidomide was later found to be efficacious in treating multiple myeloma due to its anti-angiogenic effects, and in 1965, it was trialed experimentally in the treatment of ENL with rapid resolution of the cutaneous lesions.

Experimental use for difficult-to-treat dermatologic conditions has yielded varied results, mainly in small trials, cases and series.

Clinical use in dermatology is not widespread, and the drug tends to be used after conventional treatments have failed, as second or third-line therapy.

Dermatologic prescribing

- Thalidomide is taken orally, once daily in the evening given that it causes sedation
- The initial dose depends on the condition; typically, it starts at 50–200 mg daily, but can go up to 400 mg daily in some conditions
- For cutaneous ENL, the licensed dose is 100–300 mg daily; for severe ENL, the dose may be started at 400 mg daily (once daily or in divided doses)
- Once a therapeutic effect is reached, the dose should be reduced slowly, over a period of weeks to months. However, there may be a requirement for long-term treatment, with the aim of using the lowest effective dose for maintenance therapy. Notably, the lowest effective dose may be as low as 25 mg twice weekly
- Monitoring
  - Baseline complete blood count and renal and liver function tests are recommended before treatment. Women of childbearing age need regular pregnancy tests prior to taking thalidomide and throughout the treatment course
  - Repeat blood tests at 1 and 2 months, then every 6 months
  - Close monitoring for peripheral neuropathy at each visit (every 1–2 months); patients should also be educated about signs and symptoms of neuropathy and counseled to notify prescribers immediately if these develop. Nerve conduction studies may be performed (see below)

Cautions

- Due to its major fetal toxicity, thalidomide's use is tightly regulated, and use in pregnant women is contraindicated
- Thalidomide's manufacturer, Celgene, makes it obligatory for all patients and prescribing clinicians to adhere to a special program before allowing thalidomide to be prescribed
- In the US, this is called the Thalomid REMS Program (formerly STEPS); a similar system exists in the UK called the Thalidomide Pregnancy Prevention Programme
- Contraindicated in women of reproductive potential unless they are taking precautions to avoid pregnancy. This requires the use of two methods of contraception, plus regular negative pregnancy testing before initiating and during the course of treatment
- Thalidomide is excreted in semen; male patients with a sexual partner of reproductive age should use condoms to minimize exposure

Common problems

- *Neurologic:* clinical assessments for peripheral neuropathy (a common side effect) should occur every 1–2 months. Nerve conduction studies can identify neuropathy prior to symptoms and are performed in some centers prior to treatment initiation and routinely thereafter (every 3–6 months). Other centers follow patients clinically and discontinue thalidomide if any signs or symptoms of early neuropathy develop. If undiagnosed, early peripheral neuropathy can lead to irreversible nerve damage

- Somnolence is common, requiring thalidomide to be given in the evening; dose reduction may be required

- *Hepatic derangement:* hepatocellular, cholestatic, or mixed patterns can occur, often within two months of treatment initiation. This resolves spontaneously if the drug is stopped. Any pre-existing hepatic disease should be considered carefully before commencing therapy

- *Blood disorders:* neutropenia and thrombocytopenia have been reported

- *Cardiac and vascular:* The risk of thromboembolic events (arterial and venous) and myocardial infarction is increased. Patients with a previous history of related conditions should be monitored closely; thalidomide is often avoided in patients with hypercoagulable risk factors. Bradycardia is possible; be cautious when co-prescribing drugs with similar side effects

- *Cutaneous:* Stevens–Johnson syndrome and angioedema have been described; thalidomide should be discontinued if these occur

Further reading

Faver IR, Guerra SG, Su WPD, El-Azhary R. Thalidomide for dermatology: a review of clinical uses and adverse effects. Int J Dermatol 2005; 44:61–67.

Nahmias Z, Nambudiri VE, Vleugels RA. Thalidomide and lenalidomide for the treatment of refractory dermatologic conditions. J Am Acad Dermatol 2016; 75:210–212.

Treatment pearls

- Once a therapeutic effect is reached, reduce dose to minimize risk of adverse effects

- If maintenance doses are required, the minimal efficacious dosage should be given, and further reductions should be attempted every 3–6 months

- Most patients treated with thalidomide will experience side effects; therefore, thorough patient education about potential signs and symptoms is warranted

- To ameliorate neuropathy symptoms, dose reduction may be necessary (**Table 48.1**).

- The sedative effect is exacerbated with the concomitant use of antihistamines, anxiolytics, hypnotics, antipsychotics, opiates, barbiturates, or alcohol

- Lenalidomide, a structural analogue of thalidomide also used for multiple myeloma, is now available and has little to no risk of peripheral neuropathy. Lenalidomide may prove useful in treating recalcitrant cutaneous diseases. Limited information is currently available although case reports and series on its use in dermatologic diseases exist

Table 48.1 Peripheral neuropathy: grading of severity and management. Most centers discontinue thalidomide in the setting of grade 1 or grade 2 neuropathy

Neuropathy severity	Management
Grade 1 Paraesthesia, weakness, loss of reflexes No loss of function	Monitor and consider reducing dose if symptoms worsen. Note that dose reduction may not be followed by symptom improvement
Grade 2 Function impaired, but not patient's activities of daily living	Reduce thalidomide dose or suspend treatment and monitor. Discontinue treatment if there is worsening of the neuropathy or no improvement. If neuropathy improves to Grade 1 or better, treatment can restart, if benefits outweigh the risks
Grade 3 Activities of daily living affected/impaired	Discontinue treatment
Grade 4 Disabling neuropathy	Discontinue treatment

Adapted from European Medicines Agency Evaluation of Medicines for Human Use, Assessment Report For Thalidomide Pharmion. European Medicines Agency, 2008.

Procedural dermatology

Botulinum toxin

Dermatologic indications

- Axillary hyperhidrosis
- Reduction of glabellar lines and dynamic facial rhytides
- Spasticity, strabismus, cervical dystonia, blepharospasm
- *Also used for:* Raynaud's, migraine, Frey's syndrome, chronic pain disorders

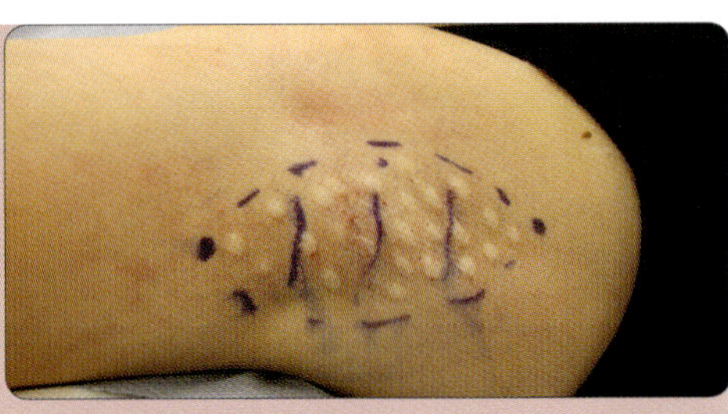

Figure 49.1 Axillary botulinum toxin.

Background

Clostridium botulinum produces 7 serotypes of botulinum toxin (A, B, C1, D, E, F, G), all of which inhibit the pre-synaptic release of acetylcholine at the neuromuscular junction.

Serotype A is licensed for use in primary axillary hyperhidrosis and glabellar rhytides and is available in three formulations: onabotulinum toxin A (Botox), abobotulinum toxin A (Dysport, Azzalure), and incobotulinum toxin A (Xeomin/Bocouture).

Botulinum toxin A inhibits the release of acetylcholine by cleaving the protein SNAP25. Cleavage prevents release of acetylcholine into the neuromuscular junction by inhibiting vesicle fusion with the presynaptic membrane.

Dermatologic prescribing

- Botulinum toxin A must be reconstituted with normal saline prior to use. Volumes used for reconstitution vary depending on formulation, treatment indication, anatomic site, and physician preference
- *Cosmetic:* Onabotulinumtoxin A and incobotulinumtoxin A are typically diluted with 2.5 mL of normal saline per 100 units, or 4 units per 0.1 mL. The recommended dilution of abobotulinum toxin A is 10 units per 0.05–0.08 mL (**Table 49.1**)
- *Facial rhytides:* the dose varies based on treatment location and patient anatomy (**Table 49.2**)

- *Hyperhidrosis:* Onabotulinumtoxin A and incobotulinumtoxin A are diluted with 5 mL of normal saline per 100 units (2 units per 0.1 mL)
- *Axillary hyperhidrosis:* 50–100 units of onabotulinumtoxin A are typically used per side for axillary hyperhidrosis. 50–100 units are frequently used per palm or sole to treat palmar or plantar hyperhidrosis. Other formulations of botulinum toxin A can also be used off-label

Cautions

- *Neuromuscular disease:* contraindicated in those with myasthenia gravis, Eaton-Lambert syndrome, peripheral neuropathy, Bell's palsy
- *Medication interactions:* caution should be used in patients taking medications that may impair neuromuscular transmission, including cholinesterase inhibitors, calcium channel blockers, aminoglycosides, quinidine
- *Pregnancy/lactation:* avoid in pregnancy as potential for risk. Safety in lactation unknown
- *Psychiatric illness:* Caution in patients with body dysmorphic disorder or unrealistic expectations

Common problems

- Pain, ecchymoses, erythema, headache
- *Uncommon:* hand weakness, ptosis, dysphagia, diplopia, swelling, compensatory hyperhidrosis and hypersensitivity

Table 49.1 Recommended dilutions of botulinum toxin used for treatment of facial rhytides

Product	Reconstitution volume	Resultant dilution
Onabotulinum toxin A (Botox)	2.5 mL per 100 unit vial	4 units/ 0.1 mL
Incobotulinum toxin A (Xeomin)	2.5 mL per 100 unit vial	4 units/ 0.1 mL
Abobotulinum toxin A (Dysport)	1.5-2.5 mL per 300 unit vial	10 units/ 0.05-0.08 mL
Abobotulinum toxin A (Azzalure)	0.63 mL per 125 unit vial	10 units/ 0.05 mL

Table 49.2 Units of botulinum toxin used for treatment of facial rhytides

Product	Glabella	Forehead	Periorbital	Nasalis	Mentalis	Perioral	Depressor anguli oris
Onabotulinum toxin A* Incobotulinum toxin A†	12.5–24[1]	10–20	15–28[3]	4–8	2–4	4–8	4–8
Abobotulinum toxin A‡	30–60[2]	25–50	30–70	10–20	5–10	10–20	10–20

FDA approved dose: 20 units[1]; 50 units[2]; 24 units[3]

*FDA approved for the treatment of glabellar and periorbital rhytids; †‡ approved for treatment of glabellar rhytides. All other treatment sites are off-label uses.

Further reading

Murray C, Solish N. Botulinum toxin injections. In: Wolverton SE (Ed). Comprehensive Dermatologic Drug Therapy, 3rd Edition. Philadelphia: Elsevier-Saunders 2012: 658–665.

Schnider P, Binder M, Kittler H, et al. A randomized, double-blind, placebo-controlled trial of botulinum A toxin for severe axillary hyperhidrosis. Br J Derm 1999; 140:677–80.

Treatment pearls

Reconstitution

- Randomized trials have found that reconstituting botulinum toxin with 0.9% saline preserved with benzyl alcohol rather than 0.9% preservative-free saline decreases injection site pain

- Reconstitution in low volumes is preferred to limit diffusion and allow for more precise treatment. Typical injection volumes are 0.05–0.1 mL per injection

- All forms of botulinum toxin A must be refrigerated prior to reconstitution except incobotulinum toxin A, which requires rotation and inversion of the bottle to ensure all toxin is reconstituted

Cosmetic use

- Different botulinum toxin formulations diffuse variable amounts. Spacing of injections and units administered will vary based on formulation and treatment site

- Consider treating only the upper portion of the frontalis, at least 2 cm above the brow, to minimize the risk of brow ptosis

- When treating the glabella, never inject lateral to the mid-pupillary line

- When treating the periorbicular region, always inject at least 0.5–1 cm away from the orbital rim to avoid diplopia. Avoid injections inferior to the zygomatic arch or while the patient is smiling to prevent ipsilateral drooping of the corner of the mouth

- Botulinum toxin is also used for treatment of rhytides on the mid and lower face, but caution should be used given the risk of affecting the muscles that control movement of the mouth and mastication. Consider one central injection if treating the mentalis to avoid asymmetry

Hyperhidrosis

- Primary hyperhidrosis: botulinum toxin should be injected intradermally to form small blebs under the skin

- Hand weakness and inability to grasp objects are risks of treatment of palmar hyperhidrosis, especially when treating over the thenar eminence

General

- Effects appear after 1–3 days, peak at approximately 2 weeks and last from 3–6 months
- Neutralizing antibodies can form to botulinum toxin, which result in shorter duration of effective therapy. In this case, switching to another formulation can be helpful

Dermatologic indications

- *Dermatologic indications:* alopecia areata, keloids and hypertrophic scars, nail psoriasis, hemangiomas, acne cysts, inflamed epidermal inclusion cysts, chondrodermatitis nodularis helicis

- *Other reported conditions:* necrobiosis lipoidica, granuloma annulare, lichen simplex chronicus, discoid lupus erythematosus, granulomatous cheilitis, hypertrophic lichen planus, lichen planopilaris, cutaneous sarcoidosis, granuloma faciale, and pyoderma gangrenosum

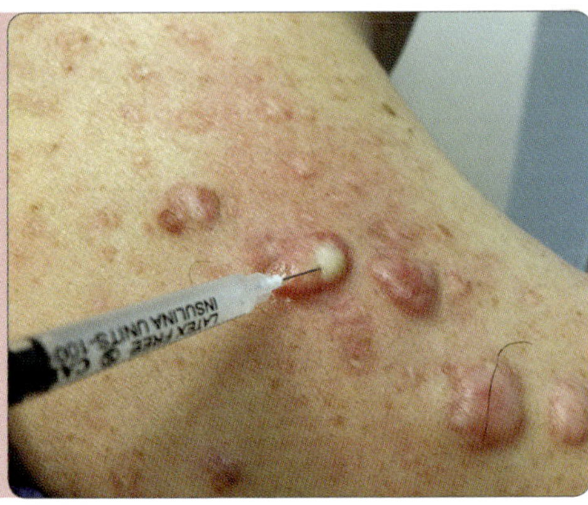

Figure 50.1 Deep infiltration of triamcinolone acetonide within a keloid scar in a patient treated for severe acne.

Background

In dermatology, corticosteroids are usually prescribed in topical form, but sometimes, when topical therapy does not produce a significant effect and systemic therapy is best avoided, steroids may be injected directly into skin lesions.

Advantages of intralesional therapies include the ability to bypass the epidermal barrier, treat conditions affecting deeper portions of the skin, and deliver a high concentration of medication in the area in need of treatment.

Although not completely understood, suppression of inflammation and reduction of collagen production are considered the major mechanisms of action for intralesional corticosteroids (see **Chapter 42**).

Dermatologic prescribing

- Triamcinolone acetonide (TA), an intermediate acting steroid, is the most commonly used intralesional steroid. TA for intralesional therapy is available in two strengths: 10 mg/mL and 40 mg/mL

- Long acting steroids such as dexamethasone and betamethasone (acetate and phosphate) are sometimes combined with TA

- The dose, concentration, and intervals between injections depends on the type, size, and severity of the lesions and on the response of previous injections (**Table 50.1**)

- Depending on the lesions to treat, dilution of TA may be required, usually with saline solution or a local anaesthetic such as mepivacaine or lidocaine

Procedure

- Clean the injection site with an antiseptic solution; TA is then usually injected using a 0.5–1.0 mL syringe with a fixed 30-gauge needle (e.g. insulin syringe)

- Other instruments such as a high-pressure injection pen (Dermojet) are also used in some countries

- The infiltration level depends on the lesion to treat. For example, intralesional steroids are injected into the mid dermis in alopecia areata and in the deep dermis (resulting in blanching of the lesion) in keloids and hypertrophic scars or hemangiomas. Subcutaneous infiltration of intralesional steroids are typically avoided due to the risk of atrophy

- Needle bevel orientation is important, upwards or downwards, depending upon where the TA needs to be deposited

Common problems

- *Pain:* this is related to lesion consistency, number of injections, and localization

Table 50.1 Recommended doses of intralesional triamcinolone for specific conditions

Condition	TA concentration (injections usually repeated every 4–8 weeks)
Scalp alopecia areata*	5 mg/mL
Eyebrow alopecia areata	2.5 mg/mL
Keloids	10–40 mg/mL
Infantile hemangioma	10–20 mg/mL
Chondrodermatitis nodularis helicis	10 mg/mL
Nail psoriasis	10 mg/mL
*A 2 × 2 cm lesion would usually require 0.25 mL	

- Infiltration of keloids and hypertrophic scars is frequently painful as the tissue is firm in consistency. After initial treatments, they soften and are easier to infiltrate, often resulting in less pain. Dilution of TA with anaesthetic may be helpful

- In alopecia areata, if plaques are numerous or large, multiple injections will be needed

- Infiltration of the palms and soles, occipital area, earlobes, and peri-nasal area may be particularly painful

- *Skin atrophy:* when injection of TA in the skin is deep and the concentration is high, an indentation limited to the injection area is common

- *Other:* telangiectasia, hyper- or hypopigmentation. Localized hypertrichosis, ulceration, and calcifications are very rare

- *Allergic reactions*: are rare, but may occur to TA itself or to benzyl alcohol contained as a preservative

- *Systemic side effects*: negligible for most dermatologic applications. Ophthalmic artery occlusion in the treatment of eyelid hemangiomas has been reported

Further reading

Firooz A, Tehranchi-Nia Z, Ahmed AR. Benefits and risks of intralesional corticosteroid injection in the treatment of dermatological diseases. Clin Exp Dermatol 1995; 20:363–370.

Jackson SM, Nesbitt LT Jr. Glucocorticosteroids. In: Bologna JL, Jorizzo JL , Schaffer JV (Eds). Dermatology, 3rd edn. Philadelphia: Elsevier-Saunders 2012: 2075–2088.

Richards RN. Update on intralesional steroid: focus on dermatoses. J Cutan Med Surg 2010; 14:19–23.

Treatment pearls

- Informed consent should be obtained as complications (both acute and delayed) and the need for repeat treatments are common

- Intralesional steroids should not be used if signs of cutaneous infection are present in the area intended for treatment

- Infiltration of firm lesions such as keloids is easier if the injection occurs during gradual needle withdrawal

- During injection, especially of firm lesions, protective eyewear and a mask are recommended to prevent splash injuries

- The practitioner should be prepared for a small amount of bleeding; apply light pressure with gauze after infiltration

- Intralesional combination therapy with steroids plus bleomycin or vinblastine may enhance the response in keloids and hypertrophic scars, but these agents are acutely painful on administration

- Cryotherapy immediately prior to infiltration of keloids may reduce pain due to the anaesthetic effect of freezing, and the induced swelling may soften the tissue to infiltrate

- Massage over the injected areas in alopecia areata may reduce the possibility of atrophy

- In selected patients, the use of topical anesthesia (e.g. topical lidocaine/prilocaine or EMLA) can be helpful for reducing the pain of intralesional injections

Iontophoresis

Dermatologic indications

- Hyperhidrosis of the hands, feet or axillae

Background

Iontophoresis describes the process in which a small electrical current is passed through the skin using a water bath.

The mechanism of action remains unclear. Some reports have suggested that hyperkeratosis develops around the sweat ducts, which reduces the flow of sweat to the surface of the skin. Other theories suggest that the electrical current alters the behavior of charged ions within the sweat glands, leading to reduced sweating.

Dermatologic use

- The current used for iontophoresis is typically 5–10 mA, which is run for 10 minutes in one direction before the polarity is reversed and run for an additional 10 minutes in the opposite direction. The size of the current is gradually increased during treatment up to a maximum of 20 mA

- The patient immerses both hands and/or both feet in water baths, usually containing normal tap water. A circuit is formed connecting the machine and both water baths, and a small electrical current is passed through the patient

- For axillary treatment, foam pads are soaked in water and held in the axillae while the current is passed through the pads and into the skin. Due to problems maintaining good contacts, axillary iontophoresis is generally less successful than hand or foot treatments

- With repeated treatments, there is a reduction in sweating in the majority of patients. However, continued treatment is needed to maintain the benefit. A variety of different treatment schedules have been described including Monday, Wednesday, Friday for 3–4 weeks as well as a regimen with treatments on days 1, 2, 7, 10, 15 and 22. A consensus on the optimal regimen does not exist, and once self-treating, patients will generally work out the treatment frequency that they need in order to control their hyperhidrosis

- Iontophoresis is available in some dermatology clinics. Patients can trial the iontophoresis for 2–4 weeks to assess response. If the treatment

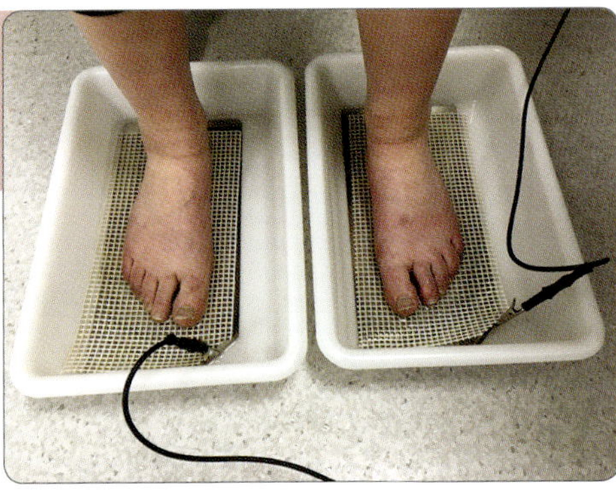

Figure 51.1 Tap water iontophoresis for the feet.

is effective, the patient will often purchase a machine for long-term treatment at home. Machines cost approximately US$600 (£400).

Additional drugs used in iontophoresis

- The water baths usually contain tap water only, which is generally effective. However, some research has been done to investigate the addition of other drugs to the water bath. A solution of an anticholinergic drug, glycopyronium bromide 0.04%, has been used, and various techniques to iontophorese botulinum toxin have been reported. There is insufficient data to know whether these techniques are superior to tap water alone

Cautions

- The hands or feet should not be removed from the water bath while the current is flowing. This results in a surge of current and can deliver a small electric shock

- Any broken areas of skin need to be covered with petroleum jelly

- Iontophoresis is contraindicated in patients with pacemakers, other implantable devices, or metal implants including joint replacements, and in pregnancy. A joint replacement is only a problem if it is in the path of the flow of current; for example, hand iontophoresis is safe with a hip replacement. Small screws at any location are not a contraindication to iontophoresis. Although no formal studies have investigated the effect of iontophoresis on intrauterine devices (IUDs), a woman with an IUD is not excluded from treatment

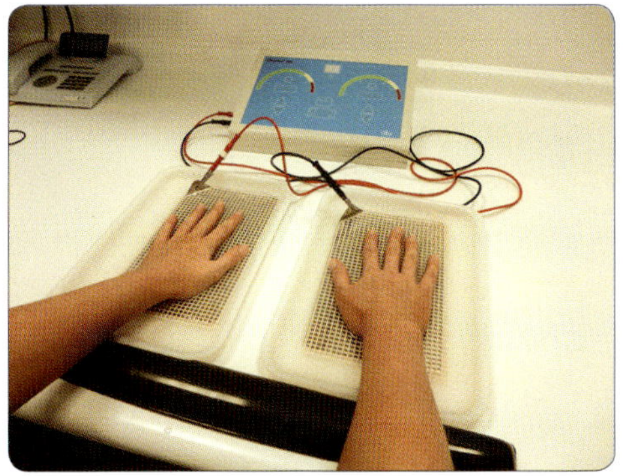

Figure 51.2 Tap water iontophoresis for palmar skin.

Common problems

- A 'pins and needles' like sensation is quite common and is usually well-tolerated. Occasionally, patients find this very uncomfortable and can only tolerate an extremely low current, resulting in a reduced chance of success
- Hand eczema can occur as a result of persistent hyperhidrosis, which can sometimes be made worse by iontophoresis. Optimizing hand eczema therapy pre-iontophoresis is recommended

Further reading

Chia HY, Tan AS, Chong WS, Tey HL. Efficacy of iontophoresis with glycopyrronium bromide for treatment of primary palmar hyperhidrosis. J Eur Acad Dermatol Venereol 2012; 26:1167–1170.

Kavanagh GM, Oh C, Shams K. BOTOX delivery by iontophoresis. Br J Dermatol 2004; 151:1093–1095.

Siah TW, Hampton PJ. The effectiveness of tap water iontophoresis for palmoplantar hyperhidrosis using a Monday, Wednesday, and Friday treatment regime. Dermatol Online J 2013; 19:14.

Laser therapy

Dermatologic indications

- Acquired vascular lesions: telangiectasias, cherry angiomas, spider angiomas, pyogenic granulomas, venous lakes, varicose veins
- Congenital vascular lesions: hemangiomas and vascular malformations including capillary malformations (port-wine stains)
- Hair removal
- Tattoo removal
- Pigment reduction
- Resurfacing of the skin

Background

LASER is an acronym for light amplification by stimulated emission of radiation.

Laser functions via the theory of selective photothermolysis: laser wavelength, pulse duration, and fluence can be used to target and confine heat to specific chromophores.

Specific skin chromophores absorb the laser light dependent upon the wavelength. Thus, different anatomical structures can be targeted, e.g. melanin, hemoglobin, water.

Cooling systems help decrease epidermal injury and subsequent adverse effects.

Dermatologic use

- Patient selection is critical and depends upon the condition being treated, skin type, presence of tan, anatomic location, and patient expectations
- It is critical to obtain a careful history from patients prior to treatment, including a history of rhytidectomy, connective tissue disorders, skin diseases that Koebnerize, or previous therapy with gold
- A history of keloid or hypertrophic scarring may require more conservative therapy
- A delay of 6–12 months should elapse after isotretinoin therapy prior to laser treatment
- Topical anesthesia may be applied 30 minutes to 1 hour prior to treatment
- Multiple treatments are often required to achieve the desired results

Vascular lesions

- Laser targets hemoglobin to heat and damage vessels
- Vessel depth, diameter, location, and distribution as well as skin type should all be considered to select laser wavelength, pulse duration, and spot size

- Caution should be observed with 1064 nm Nd:YAG lasers given their relative arterial selectivity and higher risk for scarring
- Most commonly, the 585–595 nm pulsed dye lasers are used. Other options include the 532 nm potassium titanyl phosphate (KTP), long-pulsed 755 nm alexandrite, long-pulsed 1064 nm neodymium:yttrium aluminum garnet (Nd:YAG), and intense pulsed light with appropriate filters
- Endpoints range from vessel clearance to erythema, transient purpura, and mild purpura

Pigmented lesions

- Laser targets melanin, therefore the location of the melanin (i.e. epidermal, dermal) directs laser selection
- Treatment of melanocytic nevi is generally not recommended because of the lack of histology and the unknown risks of treatment
- Dermatologic indications
- Epidermal lesions – lentigines:
  - Lasers utilized: frequency-doubled Nd:YAG (532 nm), Q-switched (QS) ruby (694 nm), QS alexandrite (755 nm)
  - Larger photo-damaged areas or many lentigines: consider treating full cosmetic unit with other modalities such as fractionated laser
  - Café-au-lait macules, ephelides may respond completely or partially and may recur
- Dermal lesions – Nevus of Ota, Nevus of Ito, dermal melanocytosis:
  - Lasers utilized: QS ruby (694 nm), QS alexandrite (755 nm). For darker skin types, consider QS Nd:YAG (1064 nm)

Tattoo removal

- Laser targets exogenous tattoo pigment (cosmetic, medical or traumatic)

- Q-switched lasers deliver nanosecond or picosecond pulses to rupture pigment-containing cells, releasing pigment that is then cleared
- Pigment particles are cleared through transepidermal elimination or lymphatic drainage
- Pigment concentration and levels within the dermis vary. Response may be difficult to predict
- Laser selection is based on the color of ink and skin type:
- Red tattoos best removed with frequency-doubled QS Nd:YAG (532 nm)
- Green tattoos best removed with QS ruby (694 nm), QS alexandrite (755 nm)
- Blue-black tattoos best removed with QS ruby (694 nm), QS alexandrite (755 nm), QS Nd:YAG (1064 nm). Black tattoos respond best to treatment
- Darker skin phototypes are best treated with QS Nd:YAG (1064 nm)

Skin resurfacing

- Treats rhytides, dyspigmentation, dermatoheliosis, skin texture and tone, surgical scars, acne scarring
- Ablative lasers:
- The target is water. The skin surface is ablated and residual thermal damage below the ablated layer leads to tissue remodeling
- Lasers utilized: carbon dioxide (CO_2) laser (10,600 nm), erbium (Er):yttrium aluminum garnet (Er:YAG) (2940 nm) or Er:yttrium scandium gallium garnet (Er:YSSG) (2790 nm) laser
- Significant recovery time is required
- Fractionated lasers:
- Create thousands of vertical columns of thermal injury per cm^2 with islands of normal tissue between; leads to healing by local remodeling. Delivered by rolling or stamping scanners
- Lasers utilized: Non-ablative fractionated devices include Er:glass (1540-1550 nm), Er:fiber (1550 nm), or Thulium fiber (1927 nm)
- Ablative fractionated devices include carbon dioxide (CO_2) laser (10 600 nm), Er:YAG (2940 nm), or Er:YSSG (2790 nm) laser
- The laser energy and density are the most important parameters for fractional devices

Cautions

- The patient, operator, and others in the treatment room must wear wavelength-specific eye protection
- Device parameter selection is crucial for treatment efficacy and to avoid complications. It is critical to adjust parameters to achieve the desired clinical endpoint
- A test site should be considered prior to full treatment to assess for adverse effects
- There is an increased risk of hypopigmentation with darker skin types, which is more common with the QS ruby laser

Further reading

Astner S, Anderson RR. Treating vascular lesions. Dermatol Ther 2005; 18:267–281.

Stewart N, Lim AC, Lowe PM, Goodman G. Aus J Dermatol 2013; 54:173–183.

Zachary C, Rofagha R. Laser therapy. In: Bologna JL, Jorizzo JL , Schaffer JV (Eds). Dermatology, 3rd Edn. Philadelphia: Elsevier-Saunders 2012: 2261–2282.

Treatment pearls

- Paradoxical darkening may occur with tattoo removal and is seen more commonly in skin-colored and cosmetic tattoos as well as with brown, yellow, and white tattoos
- Laser treatment is not recommended for allergic tattoo reactions
- Complications must be discussed before treatment and include hypo- and hyperpigmentation, textural changes, scarring, and hypersensitivity reactions
- Ablative resurfacing is the most traumatic type of laser and risks include: infections, pain, prolonged erythema, edema, delayed hypopigmentation, milia and scarring
- Areas of thinner skin (e.g. neck and chest) require less energy and density. Overlapping of the direct treatment area should be avoided, and time for cooling between passes should be allowed
- Gold intake is a contraindication to certain types of laser therapy given the risk of chrysiasis

Liquid nitrogen

Dermatologic indications

- *Benign lesions:* seborrheic keratoses, acrochordons, verrucae (viral warts), molluscum contagiosum, mucoceles, myxoid cysts, dermatofibromas, sebaceous hyperplasia, solar lentigines, angiomas
- *Precancerous lesions:* actinic keratoses, squamous cell carcinoma in situ (Bowen's disease)
- *Malignant lesions:* superficial and nodular basal cell carcinoma (only in selected cases)

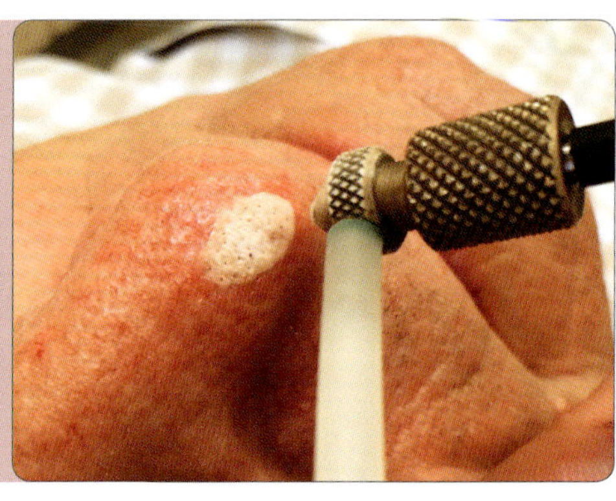

Figure 53.1 Cryotherapy of an actinic keratosis on the nasal tip.

Background

Liquid nitrogen therapy is a form of cryotherapy typically performed in an outpatient setting. It is a destructive procedure used in a wide variety of skin lesions.

A critical step in appropriate therapy with liquid nitrogen is having the correct diagnosis prior to proceeding with cryotherapy.

Mechanism of action and equipment

- The boiling point of liquid nitrogen is -196°C, making it a potent cryogenic agent. Destruction of cells by cryotherapy is believed to occur due to intracellular and extracellular changes within the cell following ice formation and damage to the cell membrane resulting in cell death
- Keratinocyte cell death will occur at approximately -50°C. Melanocyte death will occur at only -5°C, which explains why hypopigmentation frequently occurs following cryotherapy
- Application of liquid nitrogen can be performed by a Cryogun spray canister with different nozzles of varying aperture size and length, by a cotton-tipped applicator, or by cryoprobes of different sizes. The Cryogun spray is the most commonly used method. The method of liquid nitrogen application has a major influence on the extent and depth of freezing and therefore on the efficacy of treatment

Procedure

- Liquid nitrogen spray is directed toward the lesion at a distance of 1–2 mm and can be dispensed by pulses, continuously, paintbrush, or spiral method. In the UK and US, a size C nozzle is the standard

Table 53.1 Common skin lesions treated with liquid nitrogen therapy

Indication	Freezing time (seconds)	Number of freeze/thaw cycles
Viral wart (verruca)	15–30	1–2
Molluscum contagiosum	5–10	1
Acrochordon	5–10	1
Seborrheic keratosis	10–15	1–2
Sebaceous hyperplasia	5–10	1
Myxoid cyst	15–20	1
Mucocele	10	1
Dermatofibroma	20–60	1–2
Solar lentigo	3–5	1
Cherry angioma	10	1
Actinic keratosis	5–20	1
Squamous cell carcinoma in situ (Bowen's disease)	20	1–2
Basal cell carcinoma	60–90	2–3

- The duration of freezing and thawing and the number of cycles performed vary depending on the lesion to destroy (**Table 53.1**)
- Freezing of benign and precancerous lesions should include the lesion and a frozen margin of

1–2 mm. Freezing times vary based on the lesion type and thickness, but are usually shorter than for malignant lesions

- Freezing of malignant lesions should include the lesion and a frozen margin of 3–5 mm. Typically, two cycles of rapid freezing and slow thawing are recommended

Contraindications

- Skin lesions without a clear diagnosis should not be treated with cryotherapy
- Lesions that need a histopathologic sample for diagnosis (example: melanocytic nevi) should also not be treated with cryotherapy
- Avoid cryotherapy in patients with a history of cold urticaria, cryoglobulinemia, and cryofibrinogenemia should be treated with caution. In addition, caution should be employed when treating patients with a history of pyoderma gangrenosum, Raynaud's disease, or poor peripheral circulation

Cautions

- Informed consent should be obtained as need for repeat treatments as well as acute or delayed complications are common

Common problems

- *Immediate:* Headache in cranial treated areas, pain, swelling and redness, subcutaneous emphysema , vasovagal syncope, blister formation with or without haemorrhagic bullae formation
- *Delayed:* hemorrhage, infection, excessive granulation tissue, ulceration
- *Prolonged, temporary:* milia formation, hypo- or hyperpigmentation, change of sensation due to nerve injury (mainly fingers and preauricular areas)

- *Permanent:* alopecia, atrophy, keloid, scarring, hypopigmentation (especially in dark skinned patients)
- *Recurrence of the treated condition:* confirm diagnosis prior to repeat treatment

Further reading

Kuflik EG, Kuflik JH. Cryosurgery. In: Bologna JL, Jorizzo JL, Schaffer JV (Eds). Dermatology, 3rd Edn. Philadelphia: Elsevier-Saunders 2012: 2283–2290.

Unger JG, Amirlak B, Kenkel JM. Cryotherapy. Clinical Procedures Articles. New York: Medscape: Jan 29, 2015.

Abramovits W, Graham G, Har-Shai Y, Strumia R (Eds). Dermatological cryosurgery and cryotherapy, 1st Ed. London: Springer-Verlag, 2016.

Treatment pearls

- Anesthesia may be needed in children and some adults. Topical anesthesia with lidocaine/prilocaine cream may be tried initially, or if inadequate, an injected local anesthetic can be used
- Hydrating dry, scaly lesions with gauze impregnated with saline solution or water enhances the freezing process and aids in destruction of the target lesion
- The use of paracetamol or ibuprofen reduces pain during treatment. Scheduled analgesia following cryotherapy is also helpful for large or painful areas such as the fingers
- Post-treatment clobetasol propionate is sometimes used to limit blistering
- Frequent soaking with alcohol-impregnated gauze reduces swelling and blister formation of treated lesions

Photodynamic therapy

Dermatologic indications

- Lesion- and field-directed treatment for actinic keratoses, especially for multiple/confluent lesions

- Squamous cell carcinoma in situ (Bowen´s disease), especially for large plaques and those in sites of poor healing (e.g. lower legs)

- Basal cell carcinoma; ideal for superficial variants. Low risk, thin nodular BCC's may be treated if surgery is not appropriate. PDT is not appropriate for high risk BCCs (morpheaform, micronodular, ill-defined, aggressive histology)

- *Also used for:* prophylactic prevention of skin cancers, acne and other inflammatory dermatoses, refractory hand/foot and genital warts and photorejuvenation

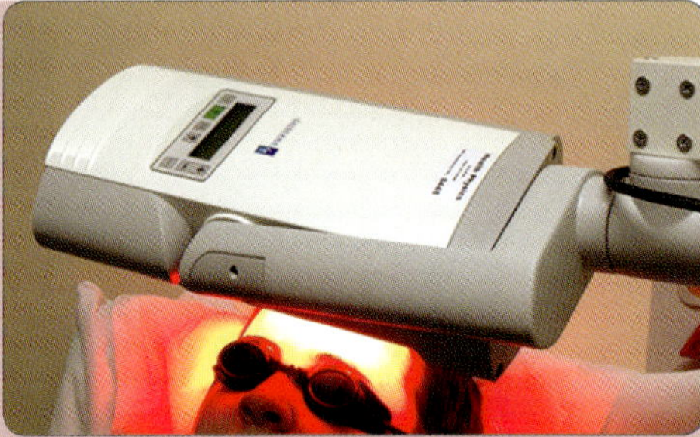

Figure 54.1 Typical PDT treatment with a red light emitting diode device is used to treat a basal cell carcinoma on the forehead.

Background

Photodynamic therapy (PDT) is a treatment that makes use of a photosensitizer, retained within the target tissue, which is activated by visible light. The light promotes a reaction involving the release of reactive oxygen species, typically resulting in the death of the target cells.

Light of an appropriate wavelength for activation of the photosensitizer is required. Red light-emitting diode devices are now the most widely used.

Three agents are currently licensed for PDT in Europe; all are recommended for use with red light sources: Methyl aminolaevulinate (MAL) is used for all above licensed indications. A nanoemulsion of aminolaevulinic acid (ALA) and a patch containing 5-ALA are both currently licensed only for the treatment of actinic keratoses.

A 20% formulation of 5-ALA is approved for actinic keratoses in a protocol that uses blue light in North America and certain other countries.

Red fluorescence can be demonstrated using a Wood's lamp following application of the photosensitizing creams and just prior to therapeutic illumination, assisting in lesion definition as well as in identifying persistent/recurrent disease that may not be clinically obvious.

PDT using MAL cream with daylight as the activating light source is as effective as standard PDT in treating thin and moderate thickness actinic keratoses on the face and scalp, and is almost painless, unlike standard PDT.

Dermatologic prescribing

- *Standard PDT:* scales and crusts are removed and then a thin layer of cream is applied to the lesions. For hyperkeratotic lesions, this may require gentle curettage with topical or local anesthetic. The area is covered with an occlusive dressing for 3 hours, then wiped clean before illuminating with red light for around 10 minutes depending on the light source used. For SCC in-situ (Bowen's) and BCCs, treatment is often repeated at 7 days

- *Daylight PDT:* a chemical sunscreen is applied to all sun-exposed areas 15 minutes before skin preparation. MAL cream is then applied to the lesions, without occlusion. Daylight exposure should begin within 30 minutes after cream application, for 2 hours

Common problems

- Pain/discomfort is commonly experienced during standard PDT, most often when treating actinic keratoses, lesions on the face or scalp, and over large treatment areas

- Various methods are used to diminish pain, including local anesthesia, cold air, and spraying the treatment site with water

- Following treatment, photosensitivity can persist for up to 48 hours; protection of the treatment site from light is advised

Further reading

Morton CA, Szeimies R-M, Sidoroff A, Braathen LR. European guidelines for topical photodynamic therapy part 1: treatment delivery and current indications – actinic keratoses, Bowen's disease, basal cell carcinoma. J Eur Acad Dermatol Venereol 2013; 27:536–544.

Morton CA, Szeimies R-M, Sidoroff A, Braathen LR. European guidelines for topical photodynamic therapy part 2: emerging indications. J Eur Acad Dermatol Venereol 2013; 27:672–679.

Morton CA, Wulf HC, Szeimies RM, et al. Practical approach to the use of daylight photodynamic therapy with topical methylaminolevulinate for actinic keratosis: a European consensus. J Eur Acad Dermatol Venereol 2015; 29:1718–1723.

Piacquadio DJ, Chen DM, Farber HF, et al. Photodynamic therapy with aminolevulinic acid topical solution and visible blue light in the treatment of multiple actinic keratoses of the face and scalp: investigator-blinded, phase 3, multicenter trials. Arch Dermatol 2004; 140:41–6.

Treatment pearls

- PDT is most suitable for patients with large and/or multiple lesions, especially in poor healing sites
- PDT is a good option for treating an entire area where multiple actinic keratoses are present, indicative of field change/carcinogenesis
- High compliance levels are achieved with PDT
- As PDT is tissue sparing and associated with a high quality cosmetic outcome, it has a place in treating lesions in cosmetically important sites
- Daylight PDT has high approval ratings from patients as it is virtually painless

Phototherapy

Dermatologic indications

- Psoriasis, atopic dermatitis, other eczematous disorders, cutaneous T-cell lymphoma (mycosis fungoides), pityriasis lichenoides chronica, vitiligo morphea, pruritus, polymorphic light eruption

Background

Ultraviolet (UV) phototherapy is used to treat a wide range of skin disorders.

Phototherapy options include: narrowband (311–312 nm) ultraviolet B (UVB), high intensity UVB (e.g. excimer 308 nm lamp) which treats small areas in patients with vitiligo or psoriasis, psoralen ultraviolet A (PUVA) photochemotherapy treatment, and less commonly, ultraviolet A1 (UVA1) which is used for morphea amongst other conditions and has the benefit of deeper penetration into the skin.

Ultraviolet B phototherapy (UVB)

- The starting dose of UVB is best determined by measuring the patient's minimal erythema dose (MED; the shortest exposure to ultraviolet light that produces barely perceptible reddening of the skin) although exposure regimens based on the patient's skin type can also be used

- Three times weekly treatment is optimal for psoriasis; twice weekly treatment is often adequate for other disorders. A typical course may last for 8-12 weeks or longer

- The dose of UVB is increased during the course of treatment to maximize effectiveness as the skin photoadapts through tanning and thickening

- The increased risk of skin cancer attributed to narrowband UVB is thought to be low

Psoralen photochemotherapy (PUVA)

- In PUVA, UVA exposure is delivered to skin following administration of a photosensitizing agent, 8 methoxypsoralen (8-MOP)

- In oral PUVA, 8-MOP is taken 2 hours before exposure (dose dependent upon body surface area)

- UVA blocking sunglasses need to be worn when outside during daylight hours on the day of psoralen ingestion to prevent retinal photodamage

- 8-MOP can sometimes induce severe nausea, in which case 5-MOP can be used

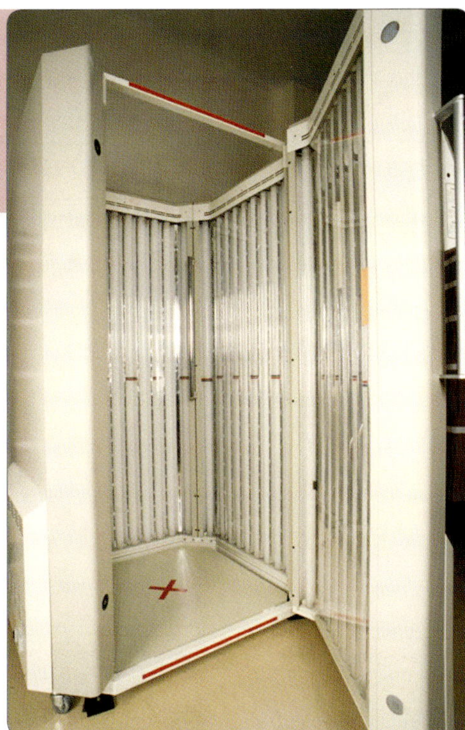

Figure 55.1 Whole body phototherapy cabinet.

- In bath PUVA (avoids nausea and ocular complications), the patient soaks in a solution of 8-MOP for 15 minutes prior to exposure (treatment of the face is not possible)

- Local immersion or application of psoralen gel can be used to treat patients with disease limited to the hands and feet

- PUVA-induced erythema is not maximal until 72 to 96 hours after exposure; therefore, treatments are given twice-weekly, usually for around 10 weeks

- The starting dose of UVA is best determined by measuring the patient's minimal phototoxic dose (analogous to MED measurement in UVB phototherapy)

- As with UVB phototherapy, the dose of UVA is increased during the course of treatment as the skin photoadapts

- A high cumulative dose of PUVA is a significant risk factor for skin malignancy. Thus, PUVA is usually reserved for patients who have failed UVB, and is rarely used in children or those with skin type I. A lifetime maximum of five courses is appropriate for most patients

- Maintenance PUVA is not recommended

Ultraviolet A1 (UVA1)

- UVA1 (340-400 nm) penetrates deeper into the dermis than UVB or UVA2 (320-400 nm) and can effect lymphocytes, fibroblasts, dendritic and mast cells

- Whole-body UVA1 lamps are cumbersome and not widely available, but smaller units can be used to treat selected areas of skin

- UVA1 has been used to treat a number of conditions including morphea, atopic dermatitis, cutaneous T-cell lymphoma and urticaria pigmentosa

Psoriasis

- Clearance of plaque-type psoriasis can be achieved with narrowband UVB in around 70% of patients

- PUVA can achieve clearance in up to 90% of patients

- UVB or PUVA can be used as single agents, or combined with topical treatments (with the exception of tacrolimus), or combined with systemic agents including acitretin, methotrexate, or biologic drugs, but not with cyclosporine or azathioprine

Atopic dermatitis

- Many patients with atopic dermatitis improve with narrowband UVB; PUVA is now rarely used to treat atopic dermatitis

- Other forms of eczema, including nummular eczema and prurigo nodularis may also respond to treatment with UVB

Polymorphic light eruption

- Narrowband UVB is helpful for many patients with polymorphic light eruption; it may prevent the rash from developing or reduce the severity

- A course of treatment, typically 12 or 16 exposures, may be given in the spring before the onset of the rash, or before a vacation where sun exposure is likely

Cutaneous T-cell lymphoma

- Patch stage cutaneous T-cell lymphoma usually responds well to narrowband UVB, with PUVA being reserved for patients with thicker plaques

Vitiligo

- Repigmentation can often be achieved with narrow-band UVB for facial and upper body vitiligo, although long courses may be required

- Repigmentation on the hands or legs is rarely seen

- PUVA is no longer recommended for vitiligo

Further reading

Zanolli M, Farr PM. Phototherapy with UVB: Broadband and Narrowband. In: Lim HW, Honigsmann H, Hawk JLM (Eds). Photodermatology. New York: Informa Healthcare 2007: 319–334.

Treatment pearls

- In all forms of phototherapy, the male genital skin should not be exposed because of an increased risk of malignancy at this site

- If the facial skin is not involved, this area should be protected with a UV-blocking visor

- Goggles are normally worn during phototherapy, but if there is eyelid involvement, treatment can be given without goggles if the patient is competent to keep the eyes closed during exposure

- Psoriasis below the knees is often resistant to phototherapy and may require additional time while standing on a slightly raised platform to move the involved area of skin away from the lower-output end of the fluorescent lamps

- Successful treatment should induce disease remission for at least 3–6 months

- Atopic dermatitis and vitiligo frequently require greater than 10 weeks of therapy

Dermatologic indications

- *Diagnosis of a rash*: it is important to be aware of which component of a rash will reveal the most informative histology. Usually, this is the most inflammatory, indurated, and/or acute component
- *Diagnosis of a lesion*: biopsy of a lesion is important when complete excision is undesirable or when histologic analysis will influence the approach to subsequent excision of the lesion

Background

Knowledge of basic surgical techniques, patient and site selection, and wound closure are important for improving skin biopsy efficiency and cosmetic outcomes as well as minimizing complications.

Site and patient preparation

- Patient history, medications, and allergies should be confirmed before surgery
- Individuals on anticoagulant therapy may need to cease treatment before the procedure or may need a monitoring test prior to surgery (refer to local guidelines); this is rarely necessary for a skin biopsy
- Consent should be obtained before commencing surgery (usually written)
- Common complications to be discussed include: infection of the wound, bleeding, and scar formation. Other site/procedure specific complications should be discussed
- Skin biopsies from non-mucosal, non-infected sites are considered as clean office-based surgery
- Apply topical antiseptic prior to the biopsy (e.g. chlorhexidine solution, povidone iodide, isopropyl alcohol, or hydrogen peroxide)
- Incisional skin biopsies are performed under local anesthesia. Inclusion of epinephrine aids hemostasis and the duration of time which the anesthesia lasts
- Preoperative oral antibiotics are not routinely recommended for skin biopsies
- Local guidelines should be referred to for patients at high risk for endocarditis, systemic infection, or those with immunosuppression

Procedure

The choice of procedure will be determined by the lesion type, its size and location, as well as the physician's experience (**Table 56.1**).

Punch biopsy

- This technique requires a cylindrical 2–6 mm in diameter (or occasionally larger) scalpel blade pushed into skin to supply a vertically oriented skin sample
- The specimen includes epidermis, dermis and some amount of subcutaneous fat

- The biopsy wound is usually primarily closed with simple suturing, providing sufficient hemostasis
- It is usually recommended to cover the biopsy site with a dressing for 48 hours

Shave biopsy

- This is a superficial skin sampling technique with a horizontal cut surface
- Tissue includes the epidermis and papillary dermis
- Saucerization is the term used for a deep shave biopsy that reaches the reticular dermis using an increased blade angulation. It is sometimes used for complete excision
- Shave biopsies are most commonly performed either with a dermablade or a scalpel blade (no. 11 or no. 15) or with scissors
- Hemostasis is achieved with electrodesiccation or by application of a styptic solution with a cotton-tipped swab to the wound bed (e.g. aluminum chloride hexahydrate or ferric subsulfate). Healing is by secondary intention with a tightly applied dressing

Incisional biopsy

- An incisional biopsy removes a wedge or a part of a larger lesion
- It provides a significant amount of tissue and is therefore the best option to sample large-sized tumors or lesions involving the subcutaneous tissue
- The procedure is similar in technique to an excisional biopsy (see **Chapter 58**)
- Tissue specimens should be placed in a specimen jar in the appropriate conditions (e.g. fresh, 10% formalin, Michel's medium), depending on the required investigation and the laboratory preference. Specimen jars should be carefully labeled with the patient's identifying data and sample description

Further reading

Darouiche RA, Wall MJ, Itani KMF, et al. Chlorhexidine–alcohol versus povidone–iodine for surgical site antisepsis. N Engl J Med 2010; 362:18–26.

Ng JC, Swain S, Dowling JP, et al. The impact of partial biopsy on histopathologic diagnosis of cutaneous melanoma. Arch Dermatol 2010; 146:234–239.

Wilson W, Taubert KA, Gewitz M, et al. Prevention of infective endocarditis: guidelines from the American Heart Association. Circulation 2007; 116:1736–1754.

Table 56.1 Biopsy site and technique selection

Lesion type	Examples	Site preferred	Biopsy technique
Tumor: - Large lesion (>1 cm diameter)	KA, large SCC or BCC, skin metastasis	Thickest portion	Incisional biopsy
- Small lesion (<1 cm)	BCC or SCC	Thickest portion	Shave or punch biopsy
- Small lesion (<1 cm)	Nevi, melanoma	Include all the lesion	Excisional biopsy
- High risk site (e.g. face)	Skin tumors (e.g. BCC)	Thickest portion	Incisional or shave biopsy
Skin eruption	Eczematous, polymorphous, urticaria, lichenoid	Most recent and representative lesion (consider multiple biopsies)	Punch biopsy
Blistering eruption	Pemphigus, bullous pemphigoid	Blister edge (H&E) Perilesional skin (DIF)	Punch biopsy
Ulcer	Vascular ulcer, tumor, pyoderma gangrenosum	Ulcer margin, to include adjacent epidermis and small amount of ulcer base	Incisional biopsy
Vascular eruption	Vasculitis, microvascular occlusion syndromes	Recent onset, avoid necrotic lesions	Punch or incisional biopsy
Nail	Melanonychia, melanoma SCC	Nail matrix Nail bed/matrix	Punch or incisional biopsy
Oral	SCC, melanoma, lichen planus	Thickest portion	Shave biopsy
Hair	Scarring or cicatricial alopecias	Active lesion, avoid scarred area	Punch biopsy aligned with the hair shafts to capture hair bulbs
Subcutaneous	Panniculitis, fasciitis	Thickest portion, most recent onset	Incisional biopsy to include large sample of subcutaneous fat

BCC, basal cell carcinoma; DIF, direct immunofluorescence; H&E, hematoxylin and eosin; KA, keratoacanthoma; SCC, squamous cell carcinoma

Treatment pearls

- The use of epinephrine (adrenaline) near terminal arterioles (e.g. fingers, toes) should be avoided

- In a widespread rash, biopsies below the knee should generally be avoided as these areas heal more slowly and are often less informative

- Scalp biopsies to confirm androgenetic alopecia generally require that the operator requests vertical and horizontal sections from the site in question and from an unaffected area (e.g. lateral scalp)

- Punch biopsy is usually inadequate for conditions in which histologic analysis of the subcutaneous fat is important (e.g. panniculitis); an incisional or wedge biopsy should be performed instead

- Biopsy of suspected leukocytoclastic vasculitis is typically uninformative when the clinical examination is classic. When IgA vasculitis is suspected, direct immunofluorescence testing for IgA deposition is warranted

- A biopsy for direct immunofluorescence should generally be undertaken in all blistering disorders, and the sample should be taken peri-lesionally

- Direct immunofluorescence in cutaneous lupus is often unhelpful because of the low specificity and sensitivity of this test

- Analysis of T-cell receptor gene rearrangement may be helpful in the diagnosis of cutaneous T-cell lymphoma (mycosis fungoides). The assay sensitivity is enhanced by sending a larger sample (6 mm) of the most inflamed area of skin on saline (fresh) for PCR

Curettage

Dermatologic indications

- Seborrheic keratoses, viral warts, skin tags, molluscum contagiosum, pyogenic granulomas, cherry angiomas, mucous cysts, sebaceous hyperplasia

- *Also used for:* Actinic keratoses and superficial basal cell carcinomas (BCCs) in low risk areas (by experienced dermatologists)

Background

Curettage is a widely used technique, mainly to treat benign lesions.

Curettage is a rapid and inexpensive procedure, which often provides reasonable cosmetic results with a low incidence of surgical complications such as infection.

Curettage allows for histopathologic examination of the surgical specimen, however, it is not an adequate technique for assessing excision margins.

The drawbacks of this technique include the time required for secondary intention healing (depending on the size and depth of the defect), the risk of pigmentary changes, and the risk of hypertrophic or depressed scaring.

Procedure

- Local anesthesia with lidocaine, typically with epinephrine, is injected

- Curettage can be performed using three techniques: scraping, scooping, or shave excision

- *Scraping:* first, the level of cleavage is identified. Traction is then applied using the thumb and index finger of the non-dominant hand. Holding the curette like a pencil with the dominant hand at an angle of no more than 30° to the skin, the lesion is scraped. Careful scraping should start at the periphery of the lesion and then move to the center to avoid damaging normal skin

- *Scooping:* this technique employs the same process as described above, but the angle of the curette is greater than 45°, causing a deeper defect. It is used for more deeply infiltrative lesions such as pyogenic granulomas

- *Shave excision:* the lesion should be grasped with toothed forceps. After identifying the correct level of cleavage, a cut should be made parallel to the skin with a sharp blade (no. 15)

- Curettage combined with electrocautery can be used by experienced dermatologists to treat

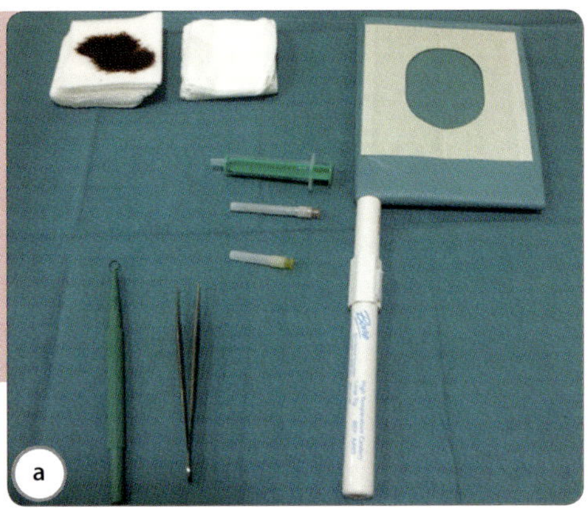

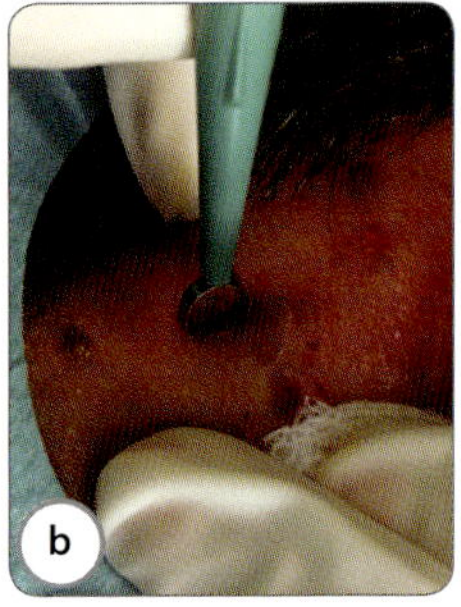

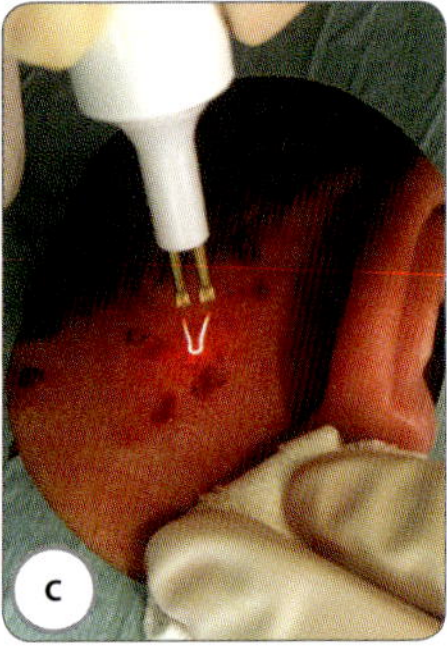

Figure 57.1
(a) Curettage material: 30 g needle, 3 mL syringe, single-use loop curette, toothed forceps, thermocautery, gauze, bandage. (b) Curettage and (c) thermocautery (coagulation).

superficial and small nodular BCCs in low risk areas (trunk and extremities). This technique usually includes three cycles of curettage and electrocautery. Occasionally thermocautery is used rather than electrocautery

- Hemostasis can be achieved by the application of direct pressure, Monsel's solution (ferric subsulfate), aluminum chloride 25%, hemostatic gelatin sponges, or with thermocautery or electrocoagulation

- Petroleum jelly or paraffin ointment should be applied to the defect and it should then be covered with a dry dressing. In large wounds, a specialized dressing should be considered in order to control the exudation and improve wound healing

Cautions

- Hyper- or hypopigmented scars, keloids and hypertrophic or depressed scars can result from this procedure. Patients with darker skin types and some anatomical areas are at an increased risk for hypertrophic scaring. These risks should be reviewed with the patient, and a consent form should be read and signed before undertaking the procedure

- In lesions in which the diagnosis is uncertain, curettage should be avoided. The specimen should always be sent for histopathologic examination

- This technique should not be utilized for lesions that require histopathologic examination of the complete lesion (e.g. a melanocytic nevus)

- Deep curettage should be avoided when the lesion is superficial as this is more likely to lead to a conspicuous scar

- Hemostasis with Monsel's solution (ferric subsulfate) may tattoo the scar. This strategy should therefore be avoided in cosmetically sensitive areas

- Although rare, wound infection can occur. If suspected, a culture of the exudate should be performed and treatment initiated

- Recurrence can occur if a lesion has not been entirely removed. The 5-year recurrence rate for BCCs in low-risk areas treated by curettage and electrocautery is 7–8% according to the British Association of Dermatologists guidelines for treatment of BCC

Further reading

Bolotin D, Alam A. Electrosurgery. In: Robinson JK, Hanke CW, Siegel DM, Fratila A (Eds). Surgery of the Skin: Procedural Dermatology, 3rd Edn. New York: Mosby-Elsevier 2015: 134–149.

Silverman MK, Kopf AW, Grin CM, et al. Recurrence rates of treated basal cell carcinomas. Part 2: Curettage-electrodesiccation. J Dermatol Surg Oncol 1991; 17:720–726

Zalla M. Basic cutaneous surgery. Cutis 1994; 53:172–186.

Treatment pearls

- Once the correct level for curettage has been identified, keep parallel to that plane

- Repeated small and superficial strokes of the curette produce the best outcome

- Dressings impregnated with topical antibiotics are not needed and are a frequent cause of contact dermatitis

Excisions

Dermatologic indications

- An excision can be used as a diagnostic tool (excisional biopsy) or as a treatment
- An excisional biopsy is commonly used for diagnosis of inflammatory diseases such as panniculitis or medium vessel vasculitis where a large and deep specimen is required
- It is also frequently used to treat skin malignancies
- Furthermore, it can be used to remove mechanically or cosmetically bothersome benign skin tumors

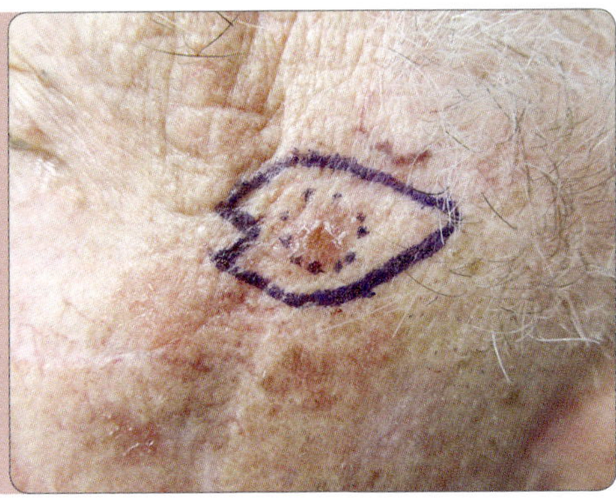

Figure 58.1 Planning of the excision of a nodular basal cell carcinoma with an ellipse and an M-plasty on the left side.

Background

Many patients visit a dermatologist with a skin tumor that warrants a simple excision.

Surgical technique

- The skin is most often disinfected with chlorhexidine gluconate (0.5%) in alcohol (70%) or chlorhexidine gluconate (1–2%) in water. Povidone–iodine solution is used less often as it causes temporary skin discoloration. There is no strong evidence that one has a better antiseptic effect than the other
- After marking the area, it is injected with a local anesthetic (e.g. lidocaine 1 or 2%, prilocaine 1 or 2%, or Xylocaine 1 or 2%). These agents can also be supplied in combination with epinephrine (adrenaline) 1:200,000, which can help to reduce peri-operative bleeding
- The scalpel is oriented vertically to the skin and the first incision is made to the level of the subcutaneous fat. Most often, an ellipse of skin is removed
- Hemostasis is achieved, typically using electrocautery
- Undermining of the wound edges decreases tension. Undermining is normally performed in the plane of the subcutaneous fat
- Subcutaneous absorbable sutures (e.g. Vicryl, Monocryl, PDS, Dexon or Polysorb) are placed to approximate the wound edges
- The skin is closed by transcutaneous or intracutaneous sutures. For transcutaneous closures, non-absorbable sutures are used (nylon [Ethilon], polypropylene [Prolene, Surgipro] and polyester [Mersilene, Dacron]). Examples of intracutaneous sutures include monofilament absorbable (Monocryl), copolymer absorbable (Vicryl) and non-absorbable sutures (Prolene)

Cautions

- The risk of intra or postoperative bleeding is increased in patients on anticoagulation. However, anticoagulants generally do not need to be stopped before a simple excision. The risk should be judged on a case-by-case basis
- With modern implantable devices and pacemakers, bipolar coagulation is unlikely to cause problems. If the practitioner is at all unsure, they should discuss this with the cardiology team or avoid electrocautery altogether
- The operating dermatologist must be familiar with the local anatomy, including what structures (arteries, veins and nerves) are present in the area to be excised
- Skin markers should be used to plan the excision. An ellipse should follow the relaxed skin tension lines
- Hypertrophic scars are more common in particular sites, such as the upper chest or back. Predisposed patients will often have problems with further surgeries
- Pregnancy and lactation: local anesthetics can cross the placenta but are generally safe to use in small volumes. Epinephrine (adrenaline) should be avoided
- Smoking delays wound healing and increases the risk of local skin necrosis
- Traction must be avoided on functional structures such as the eyelid and nasal ala

Common problems

- Every excision will result in scar formation. It will be more or less pronounced depending

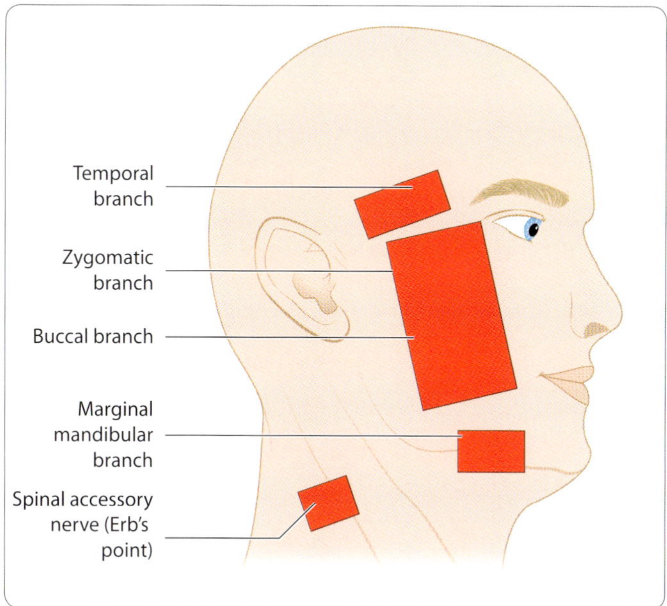

Figure 58.2 Facial nerve danger areas.

on the location, size of the lesion, and patient characteristics

- Although major complications are rare in dermatologic surgery, a patient should be pre-operatively informed and consented regarding the low rate of post-operative infection, hemorrhage, and other risks

- Damage to small sensory nerves may occur, causing areas of numbness. In facial danger zones (temporal area, jaw), motor nerves can be injured

- Excessive wound tension leading to impaired blood supply can cause necrosis

Further reading

Brown DG, Wilkerson EC, Love WE. A review of traditional and novel oral anticoagulant and antiplatelet therapy for dermatologists and dermatologic surgeons. J Am Acad Dermatol 2015; 72:524–534.

Cordoro KM, Russel MA. Minimally invasive options for cutaneous defects: secondary intention healing, partial closure, and skin grafts. Facial Plast Surg Clin N Am 2005; 13:215–230.

Hudson DA. Achieving an optimal cosmetic result with excision of lesions on the face. Ann Plast Surg 2012; 68:320–325.

Treatment pearls

- The ratio of width versus length of an ellipse is traditionally 1: 3. In practice, however, this rule may be adjusted

- A benign tumor can be excised without a surgical margin. Surgical margins are necessary in malignant tumors and are dependent on the type and size of the tumor and on whether it is a primary or a recurrent tumor

- The normal depth of a skin excision is into the subcutaneous fat. Melanoma excisions typically extend to the fascia. On the scalp, the subgaleal plane is an ideal plane for surgery as it is a relatively avascular area

- An M-plasty will reduce the length of a scar

- Not every excision needs to be closed with sutures. For example, healing by secondary intention produces very good results in concave areas of the face

Mohs micrographic surgery

Dermatologic indications

- Mohs micrographic surgery (MMS) is typically employed for tumors which have a tendency to demonstrate subclinical spread or for tumors at critical anatomical locations
- Basal cell carcinomas (BCCs) are appropriate for MMS in the following settings:
  - Tumors with ill-defined margins
  - Infiltrative, morpheaform, micronodular growth patterns
  - Tumors arising at critical sites (periocular skin, nose, lips, ears, temples)
  - Recurrent or incompletely excised tumours
  - Tumors on the head and neck in young patients
  - Large tumors (>2 cm in diameter)
- Other tumors for which MMS may be indicated include:
  - Squamous cell carcinoma
  - Lentigo maligna
  - Sebaceous carcinoma
  - Atypical fibroxanthoma
  - Dermatofibrosarcoma protuberans
  - Microcystic adnexal carcinoma

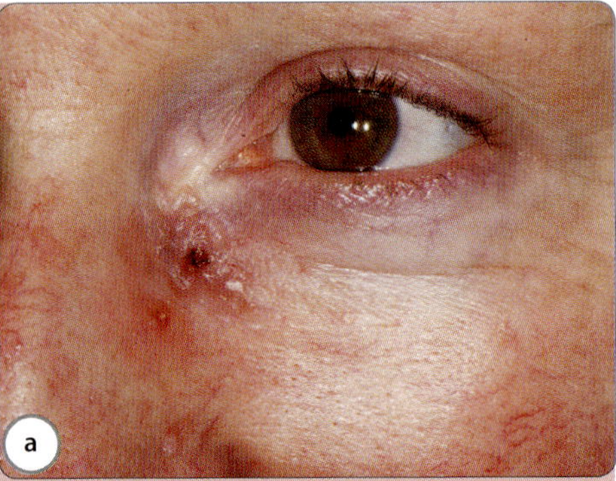
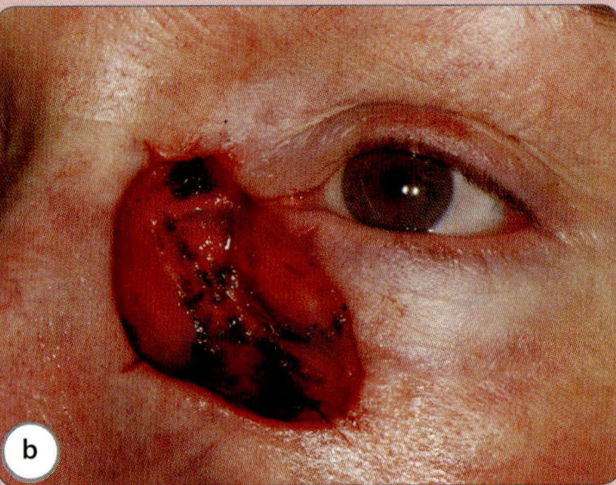

Figure 59.1 A basal cell carcinoma which exhibited a significant degree of subclinical spread before (a) and after (b) MMS.

Background

Mohs micrographic surgery (MMS), is a specialized method of surgical excision invented by Dr Frederic Mohs. It is generally performed under local anaesthesia. Mohs fellowship training is the gold standard for performing MMS. MMS aims to deliver the highest cure rates while allowing for tissue preservation.

MMS differs from standard excision by allowing for histologic examination of 100% of mapped surgical margins. High cure rates are achieved because the histology is examined intraoperatively to confirm clearance. Tissue preservation is possible because narrow excision margins can be taken given that histologic confirmation of tumor clearance is part of the procedure.

MMS is ideal for sites at higher risk of recurrence or where tissue preservation is important, such as the periocular skin, nose, lips, and ears.

Procedure

- After excision of the tumor with narrow margins, the wound base and walls are removed ('saucerization excision') and sent for cryosectioning so that 100% of the margins can be examined
- The margins are color coded so that the surgeon can re-excise only the margins where there is evidence of incomplete tumor removal. Each excision is known as a 'stage'
- This is repeated until negative tumor margins are achieved and typically takes one to three stages
- Repair of the wound/reconstruction may then be undertaken knowing that tumor clearance has been achieved

Cautions

- Informed consent should be obtained and patients warned that excision of their tumor may result in an unpredictable defect size
- Although recurrence is rare following MMS, it not impossible and patients should be advised of this risk. In particular, recurrent tumours are significantly less likely to be cured with Mohs surgery

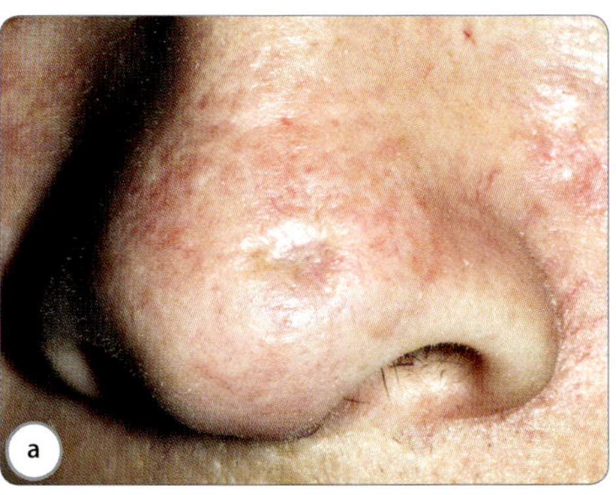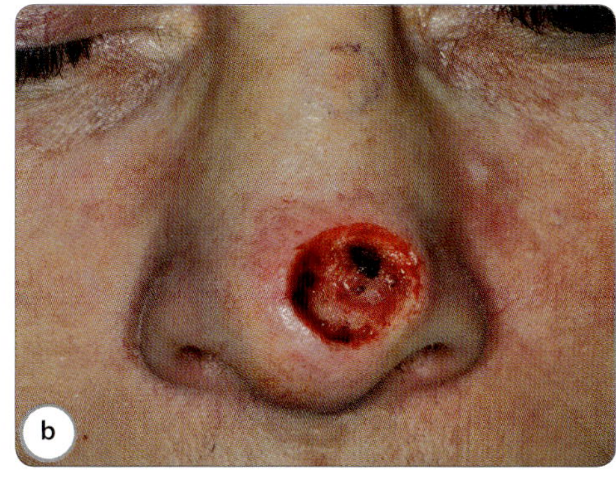

Figure 59.2 Basal cell carcinoma on the nasal tip (a) removed by Mohs technique (b).

- It is not possible to process bony tissue using MMS
- The complications of Mohs surgery are largely the same as those associated with dermatologic surgery in general

Further reading

British Association of Dermatologists Working Party on Setting Standards for Mohs Micrographic Surgery Services. Recommendations of the British Society for Dermatological Surgery and British Association of Dermatologists. London: BAD, 2011.

Brodland DG, Amonette R, Hanke W, Robbins P. The history and evolution of Mohs micrographic surgery. Dermatol Surg 2000; 26:303–307.

Leibovitch I, HuigolSC, Selva D, et al. Cutaneous squamous cell carcinoma treated by Mohs micrographic surgery in Australia. Experience over 10 years. J Am Acad Dermatol 2005; 53:253–260.

Muller FM, Dawe RS, Moseley H, et al. Randomized comparison of Mohs micrographic surgery and surgical exicision for small nodular basal cell carcinoma: tissue sparing outcome. Dermatol Surg 2009; 35:1349–1354.

Van Loo E, Mosterd K, Krekels GA, et al. Surgical excision versus Mohs micrographic surgery for basal cell carcinoma of the face: a randomised Clinical trial with ten year follow up. Eur J Cancer 2014; 50:3011–3020.

Treatment pearls

- Wounds resulting from MMS may be managed by second intention wound healing
- Reconstruction of certain anatomical sites may be best achieved by working jointly with other disciplines (e.g. oculoplastic surgery)
- Fixed tissue MMS ('slow Mohs') may be preferable in selected tumors such as lentigo maligna, DFSP, and other rare skin cancers where histopathologic interpretation is more challenging. The process may take a week or more
- Adequate training in MMS is fundamental to achieving high cure rates. Mohs fellowship training is therefore of fundamental importance

Surgical complications (management)

Background

- Surgical procedures should be considered a partnership with the patient and result in a dialogue regarding the benefits, risks, and potential outcomes
- Managing patient expectations and minimizing risks are paramount
- A procedure the surgeon considers an excellent outcome may be perceived negatively by the patient

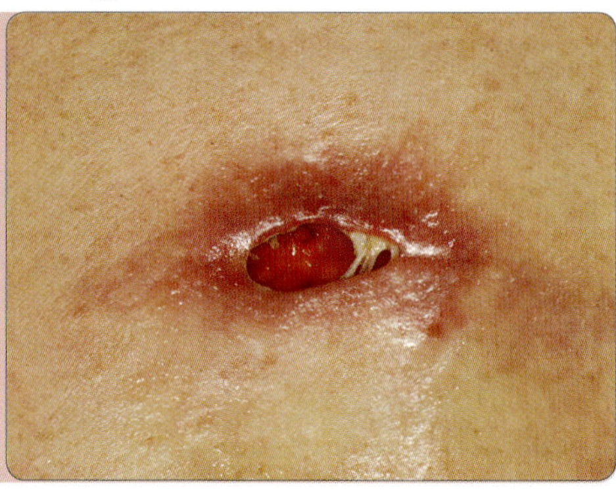

Figure 60.1 Wound dehiscence.

Pre-operative considerations

Patient education and informed consent

- Patient identifiers must be checked and the surgeon should be aware of any co-morbidities, medications, and allergies
- Confirmation of the site is vital. The procedure and the size of the resultant scar should be discussed. Use of a mirror and/or annotation of clinical notes with illustrations may be necessary
- Consent must be obtained for bleeding, hematoma, scar, pain, infection, numbness, weakness, incomplete excision, and recurrence. The likelihood of these risks will depend on the surgical site and the procedure planned

Operator safety and risk management

- The surgeon must have a trained assistant(s) as well as appropriate equipment, instruments and lighting
- A surgical cap, mask and eye protection are essential and surgical scrubs are recommended
- Both the patient and surgeon should be positioned comfortably
- Adherence to aseptic technique is critical
- The surgeon should be familiar with local risk management policies and guidelines

Intraoperative complications

- *Allergy to local anaesthetic (LA):* is a rare complication, but if present or suspected, further investigation may be necessary before proceeding to treatment. Other causes of hypotension (e.g. vasovagal syncope) should be considered
- *Pain*: LA is painful to administer. This can be minimized by using a narrow gauge needle (30 G), infiltrating slowly, using a regional nerve block, distracting the patient, and maintaining a professional controlled approach that fosters confidence
- *Bleeding*: anticoagulants increase the risk of intra- and post-operative bleeding; decisions regarding stopping anticoagulation are patient specific. Hematologic disorders may increase bleeding, and appropriate measures should be taken. Most operative bleeding is easily managed by electrocoagulation or ligation of larger vessels
- *Vasovagal episodes*: vasovagal syncope should be identified quickly and managed appropriately. If a patient loses consciousness during a procedure, immediate assistance should be requested and resuscitative procedures initiated. A well-maintained crash cart/trolley should always be available
- *Damage to nerves:* anatomical knowledge is critical to avoid inadvertent nerve injury. Damage to small cutaneous nerves may result in temporary dysesthesia, while damage to motor nerves may result in permanent muscle paralysis in the area of the nerve's distribution

Postoperative complications

- Post-procedural information allows the patient to anticipate and manage minor complications

Early complications

- *Bruising and swelling*: bruising may be dramatic even with minor procedures at certain sites, such as the forehead and nasal dorsum, where bilateral periocular bruising is common
- *Bleeding*: minor postoperative bleeding will usually respond to 15–20 minutes of local pressure. Pressure dressings for 2–3 days

postoperatively may be useful. Persistent postoperative bleeding requires urgent attention, wound assessment, and appropriate management

- *Hematomas*: hematomas present with pain and enlarging swelling around the wound caused by bleeding into the wound cavity. Small hematomas may respond to local pressure, while larger hematomas can lead to wound dehiscence, tissue necrosis, and wound infection. They may require surgical exploration and evacuation

- *Wound dehiscence*: when a wound dehiscence occurs within the first 48 hours, it may be re-sutured. Otherwise, healing via second intention is usually recommended

Late complications

Infection

- Infection should be suspected in the presence of edema, tenderness, erythema, increased warmth, and purulent discharge. Commonly isolated organisms are *Staphylococcus aureus* and *Streptococcus*

- Wound swabs should be taken for culture and sensitivity (C&S)

- Antibiotic choices include cephalosporins, clindamycin, erythromycin, floxacillin, amongst

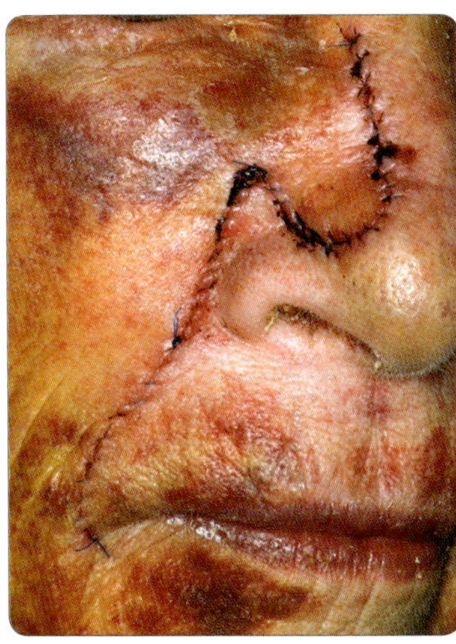

Figure 60.2 Extensive bruising may occur in some patients.

others. *Pseudomonas* should be considered in a surgical site infection of the ear

- Non-bacterial causes of infection including herpes simplex virus (HSV) should be considered

- *Infection rates:* these are operator- and procedure-specific. Studies report rates of around 1.3–2.3%. Higher rates have been described at sites including the ears, skin flexures, and legs

- *Surgery specific risk factors for infection:* use of excessive suture material, reaction to buried sutures, wound closure under excessive tension, overuse of electrocoagulation of the wound bed, and hematoma formation

- *Risk factors for postoperative infection:* obesity, immunosuppression, smoking, and diabetes. There may be increased risk in those colonized with *S. aureus* and MRSA

- *Use of antibiotic prophylaxis:* this depends on the above factors, the surgical site, and the presence of ulceration and/or crusting of the preoperative site. A preoperative swab for C&S should be considered

Scarring

- Reduction of wound tension through the use of subcutaneous sutures may reduce the risk of scar stretch. Scars should be placed parallel to relaxed skin tension lines when possible

- Keloid scars are more common in skin types V-VI, young people, and patients with a past history of keloid scarring. Keloid-prone sites include the upper chest, upper back, shoulders, upper arms, and ears

Further reading

Bordeaux JS, Martires KJ, Goldberg D, et al. Prospective evaluation of dermatologic surgery complications including patients on multiple antiplatelet and anticoagulant medications. J Am Acad Dermatol 2011; 65:576–583.

Brown SM, Oliphant T, Langtry J. Motor nerves of the head and neck that are susceptible to damage during dermatological surgery. Clin Exp Dermatol 2014; 39:677–682.

Futoryan T, Grande D. Postoperative wound infection rates in dermatologic surgery. Dermatol Surg 1995; 21:509–514.

Goodman GJ. Treating scars: addressing surface, volume and movement to optimize results: part 1: Mild grades of scarring. Dermatol Surg 2012; 38:1302–1309.

Dermatologic indications

- Dressings: leg/pressure ulcers, surgical wounds, blistering conditions (e.g. bullous pemphigoid), toxic epidermal necrolysis (TEN)
- Compression bandages: leg ulcers (venous, mixed), stasis dermatitis, lymphedema, edema secondary to venous hypertension, inflammation, resolving cellulitis

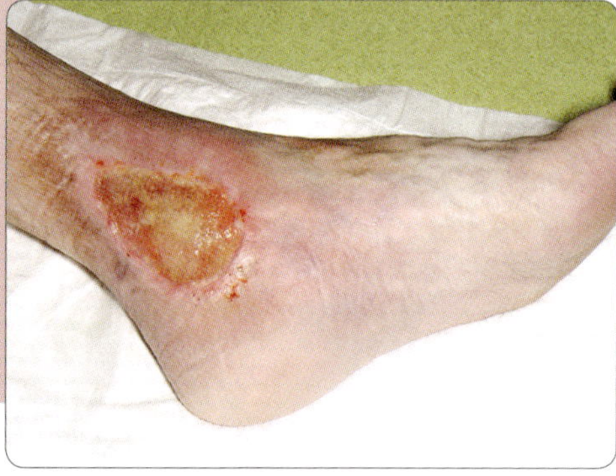

Figure 61.1 Venous ulcer.

Background

Dressing choice depends on a number of factors including the presence of infection, slough and/or necrosis, degree of exudate, and condition of surrounding skin.

The ideal dressing maintains a moist environment for optimum wound healing.

Wounds may be debrided manually if necessary or with larvae, but hydrogels and hydrofibers facilitate autolytic debridement.

Assessment of leg ulceration includes determining likely etiology, risk factors, and co-morbidities (previous DVT, varicose veins, diabetes, hypertension, smoking history). Measurement of the ankle brachial pressure index (ABPI) is helpful.

Adequate compression is essential for the treatment of venous leg ulcers. Optimization of glycemic control is critical for diabetic patients with ulcers. Arterial disease should be assessed by a vascular surgeon for the consideration of angioplasty or bypass surgery.

Dermatologic prescribing

Dressings

- *Low-adherent dressings:* e.g. Atrauman (neutral triglycerides), Mepitel (silicone). Widely used dressings including for surgical wounds. Silicone products are non-adherent and most useful for painful wounds or TEN
- *Hydrogels:* e.g. Actiform cool. These dressings donate fluid, hydrating and debriding wounds. They are useful for dry necrotic wounds (provide a moist environment) and for sloughy ulcers (facilitate debridement). The dressings turn into a gel so a secondary dressing is required
- *Hydrofibres:* e.g. Aquacel. These dressings absorb exudate and form a gel. They are good for sloughy wounds requiring debridement or for those with high exudate

- *Superabsorbent dressings:* e.g. KerraMax and Sorbion sana (polyacrylate polymers). These products wick fluid away from wounds and are a significant advance for highly exudative wounds
- *Hydrocolloids:* e.g. Granuflex. These promote healing of small wounds such as pressure sores. They can be applied over topical steroid for treatment of overgranulation, lichen planus, or lichen simplex chronicus
- *Foams:* e.g. Allevyn. These are useful to provide extra padding. They absorb some fluid, but do not remove it from the skin surface, so there is a risk of maceration
- *Alginates:* e.g. Sorbsan (calcium alginate). These are highly absorbent dressings for highly exudative wounds and for packing cavities. A secondary dressing is required
- *Antimicrobial dressings:* Suitable for highly exudative wounds at risk of colonization. Examples include Aquacel Ag containing silver and Inadine and Iodoflex, which contain iodine. Charcoal impregnated dressings may reduce odor (e.g. CarboFLEX). There are a range of products containing Manuka honey (Activon) that have antiseptic properties
- *Paste bandages:* e.g. Zipzoc (medicated rayon stockings) are used for eczema, in particular for stasis dermatitis (venous eczema). They provide a barrier to prevent scratching, improve lichenification, and aid absorption of creams/ointments. They are impregnated with 20% zinc oxide ointment and are worn under a tubular bandage or compression dressing (depending on clinical need)
- *Tubular bandages:* e.g. Tubifast, Clinifast. These are ideal for dressing retention and protecting clothes

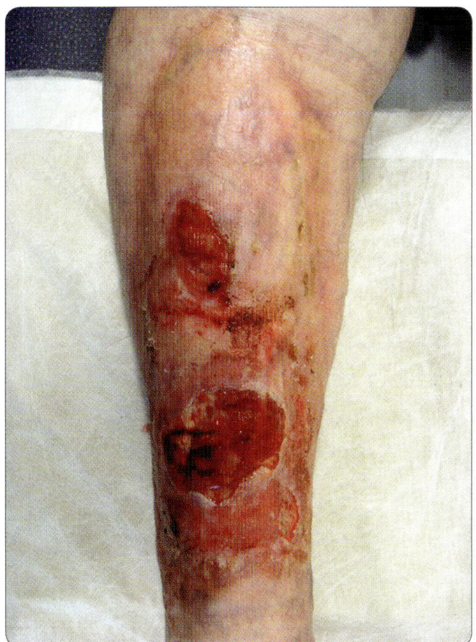

Figure 61.2 Two areas of ulceration within a plaque of necrobiosis lipoidica on the anterior shin of an elderly woman. Necrobiosis lipodica is very prone to poor healing and ulceration. This case required topical steroid treatment followed by prolonged protection with dressings to achieve full healing.

Compression bandaging

- Compression bandages are used to treat and prevent leg ulcers, edema, and lymphedema if the ABPI >0.8. These must be applied by someone with expertise. The following layers are applied (on top of any emollients/primary dressings):

  - Tubular bandage (e.g. Clinifast) to keep primary dressings in place

  - Padding layer (e.g. Softban) to shape limbs and provide protection

  - Short stretch bandage (e.g. Actico, 40 mmHg; or Elset, 15-20 mmHg). Different application techniques are required, for example Actico should be applied with 100% stretch and 50% overlap

- Compression hosiery (e.g. Activa, Mediva). Grades 1 to 3 are available. These are ideal to wear after a venous ulcer has healed and/or for the treatment and prevention of edema. The grade advised depends on the underlying problem and dexterity of the patient. For example, a patient who has had a DVT should wear the highest grade of compression they can tolerate to improve venous return. There are versions such as

Juxtafit (for edema) and Juxtacure (for sustained pressure) now available which are easier to apply, but less discreet. These are useful for elderly patients with limited mobility

Common problems

- Prolonged usage of a hydrocolloid may result in over-granulation. Therefore, wounds should be frequently reassessed, changing the dressing if necessary

- A dressing which does not adequately absorb exudate can result in maceration. Select the correct dressing in order to protect the surrounding skin

- Contact dermatitis should be considered if there is a clear cut off of eczema where bandages or dressings have been, or in stasis dermatitis (venous eczema) when there is a poor response to treatment

- A common cause of leg ulcers being slow or failing to heal is inadequate compression

- An incorrect choice of dressing can lead to wound adherence. For example, if an alginate is applied to a dry wound, fibers may be retained, providing a medium for colonization

Further reading

Menaker GM, Mehlis SL, Kasprowicz S. Dressings. In: Bolognia JL, Jorizzo JL , Schaffer JV (Eds). Dermatology, 3rd Edn. Philadelphia: Elsevier-Saunders 2012: 236–237.

National Institute for Health and Care Excellence. NICE Clinical Knowledge Summaries: Leg ulcer – venous. London: NICE, 2016. http://cks.nice.org.uk/leg-ulcer-venous (last accessed 21 July 2016).

Treatment pearls

- The correct time to change dressings or bandages is when there is leakage, odor, or pain

- A moist environment is optimal for healing, except in cases of cutaneous vasculitis. In vasculitis, wounds should be kept dry, allowing healing underneath before the eschars fall off

- In stasis dermatitis (venous eczema), the eczematous process needs to be treated with topical corticosteroids in conjunction to treating the increased pressure and edema from venous hypertension with compression

- Long term compression may prevent venous ulcers in patients with a previous DVT

Disease index

Note: Page numbers in **bold** or *italic* refer to tables or figures respectively.

Venous leg ulcers 136, *136*
Verrucae 32, 120, **120**
Viral warts 32, **120,** 128
Viral warts, resistant 40
Vitiligo 16, 125
Vitiligo morphea 124
Vulvar intraepithelial neoplasia (VIN) 30

W
Wegener's granulomatosis 84

X
Xeroderma pigmentosum 102
Xerosis *28,* 28–29
X-lined ichthyosis 50

Z
Zoster (Shingles) 73

Treatment index

Note: Page numbers in **bold** or *italic* refer to tables or figures respectively.